GET OFF MEDS

LOSE WEIGHT

HEAL DEPRESSION

DEDICATED TO MY MOTHER, WHO LOST HER LIFE TO
CANCER, AFTER DOING EVERYTHING THE DOCTOR ORDERED

PAULIE FROM OPTIMUM SOULS

PRESENTS

THE OPTIMUM 28

TABLE of CONTENTS

WELCOME TO THE OPTIMUM 28

Welcome, Optimum Souls! This is your wake-up call. It's time to take control of your health and transform your life. I know this because I was once where you are. Ten years ago, I suffered from leaky gut and acid reflux, and after seeing several doctors, none of them could diagnose me. They simply prescribed me multiple medications for life. That was the moment I realized that the medical industry didn't have the answers I was looking for.

I took it upon myself to learn about the human body and nutrition, and as I began to heal, I realized that big healthcare isn't in the business of healing us. I felt like I had unlocked a superpower, and I wanted to share my knowledge with the world. So, I created Optimum Souls, with the goal of helping people get off medication, lose weight, and heal from depression. I've created this 28-day challenge to help as many people as possible. I believe in you, and I know you can do this!

Before we begin, let's talk about what you'll need to succeed. First, choose a day to start the challenge. It's important to have at least the first three days off from work and stress because without sugar, your body will go through what's called the keto flu. This is your body's way of adjusting to a low-carb, high-fat diet. During this time, your body is going through sugar withdrawal and may try to convince you to go back to sugar. Don't give in! Stick with it, and you'll start to see the benefits.

Now, let's address some common misconceptions about diet and health. First of all, a low-fat diet isn't necessarily healthy. In fact, research has shown that saturated fat won't make you fat or lead to heart disease. Additionally, meat does not cause cancer, and does not raise cholesterol. It's important to change your mindset about these topics if you want to succeed. Fatty meat is healthy and will help heal your body, and salt is not bad for you. Also grass fed butter is very healing for the body.

It is a common occurrence for people to be misled and lied to throughout their lives. This can happen through a variety of means, such as propaganda, misinformation, and societal conditioning. Many people are taught from a young age to accept certain beliefs or ideas without questioning them, leading them to carry these beliefs throughout their lives. However, in order to truly change and grow, it is essential to question these beliefs and start over with a new perspective.

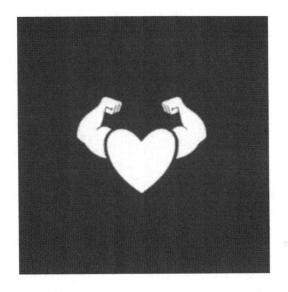

FAT DOES NOT MAKE YOU FAT

MEAT DOES NOT RAISE CHOLESTEROL

CARBS ARE NOT ESSENTIAL

SALT IS GOOD FOR YOU

SUGAR CAUSES INFLAMMATION

EGGS ARE HEALTHY

SATURATED FAT IS NOT BAD

GRAINS ARE NOT HEALTHY

LOW-FAT FOODS ARE BAD FOR YOU

VEGETABLE OIL IS BAD FOR YOU

LOW CARB DIETS ARE NOT DANGEROUS

BREAKFAST IS NOT THE MOST IMPORTANT MEAL

THE PROCESS OF CHANGE

To begin the process of change, it is important to recognize that the beliefs and ideas we hold may not be entirely accurate. We have all been influenced by external factors, such as our upbringing, culture, and education, which can lead us to accept certain ideas without questioning them. In order to break free from these influences, it is necessary to challenge our preconceived notions and examine them critically.

Starting over can be a difficult and uncomfortable process, as it requires us to confront the possibility that we have been wrong about certain things. However, it is also an opportunity to learn and grow in new ways. By approaching the world with an open mind and a willingness to learn, we can discover new ideas and perspectives that we may have never considered before. Ultimately, it is through this process of re-examining our beliefs and starting over that we can become more enlightened and better equipped to navigate the complexities of the world around us.

While it's important to have a support system and seek guidance from others, ultimately, the responsibility for change and self-improvement lies with the individual. I am going to just tell you now that you will have zero support from your friends and family. They will not change their habits around you. Waiting for someone else to help or change you is not only ineffective, but it also places your happiness and well-being in someone else's hands, rather than taking ownership and control of your life.

Only you can truly understand your thoughts, feelings, and motivations, and it's up to you to take action towards achieving your goals and making positive changes in your life. Societal beliefs can influence our behavior and beliefs, but it's ultimately up to us to choose how we respond and move forward. Moreover, the process of self-help and personal growth requires self-reflection, honesty, and dedication. It's not an easy or quick process, and it often requires making uncomfortable changes and facing our fears and vulnerabilities. However, the rewards of self-improvement and self-empowerment are immeasurable, leading to a greater sense of fulfillment, self-confidence, and overall happiness.

I want you to know that you are capable of achieving this. Sometimes, the hardest part can be breaking free from old beliefs that are holding us back. It can be tough to let go of what we've always known and embrace change, but I'm here to help guide you through the process.

Let's take a moment to imagine your future. Where do you see yourself in five years? What does your ideal life look like? Now, let's work together to make that vision a reality. In just 28 days, you can make some changes that will have a big impact on your health and your future.

And the best part? You don't have to sacrifice anything to make these changes. In fact, by adopting a new mindset and embracing this lifestyle, you'll be doing yourself a huge favor. You deserve to be happy, fulfilled, and living your best life.

TAKE EVERYDAY

(with food)
VITAMIN D3 10,000 IU
VITAMIN K2 100 mcg
(empty stomach)
MAGNESIUM GLYCINATE 450 MG

It is commonly believed that people are resistant to change, and studies have shown that approximately 80 percent of people never change. This means that despite the efforts of friends, family, or even professionals, a significant number of people are unwilling or unable to modify their beliefs, attitudes, or behaviors.

One reason why many people resist change is that they are comfortable with the status quo. Humans have a natural tendency to seek stability and predictability in their lives, and any disruption to this sense of stability can be unsettling. This is why people often prefer to stick to familiar routines and ways of doing things, even if they are not particularly satisfying or productive.

Personal growth and addiction recovery often require a significant shift in one's attitudes, beliefs, and behaviors. It is widely recognized that these changes can be challenging, requiring a great deal of effort, persistence, and courage. While it may be tempting to rely on others for support and motivation, the reality is that change ultimately comes from within.

As much as one may want to help others change, it is important to recognize that change is a personal decision that can only be made by the individual themselves. The proverbial saying "you can lead a horse to water, but you can't make it drink" rings true in this context. I am bringing you to the water, I am offering guidance and support, but only you can start drinking.

It is not uncommon for friends and family members to become frustrated and even desperate when attempting to help their loved ones change. The process of trying to change someone else can be emotionally draining, especially when it seems like no progress is being made. It can be disheartening to watch someone continue down a destructive path, despite one's best efforts to intervene.

BACON IS HEALTHY

GRASS FED BUTTER IS GOOD FOR YOU

EGGS LOWER CHOLESTEROL

DON'T LIKE SALADS OR VEGGIES?

There is nothing wrong with omitting the salad and vegetable components from the recipes I have included for this challenge, as they are not essential to meet the requirements. Rather, focus on incorporating the meat, fat, and butter as your primary sources of nutrition. If desired, feel free to increase the quantity of meat and reduce or eliminate the plant-based ingredients.

CHOOSE A DAILY ACTIVITY

This challenge will require you to do 2 physical activities everyday. One of them is a 10 minute or longer walk directly after your first meal and you will choose the second activity. It can be anything you want! Keep it easy so you do not get intimidated. When I first started this lifestyle, I was doing only 3 push ups a day. Some examples are squats, pull ups, push ups, or jumping jacks. Make it easy!

MAKE FAT YOUR NEW SUGAR

The first step to desiring fat over sugar is to increase your fat intake. Your body is accustomed to using sugar for energy, so it may take some time to adjust to using fat as your primary energy source. As you incorporate more fat, you will feel more full, which will reduce your cravings for sugar.

Shifting your preferences towards fats can be obtained when you stop sugar. Sugar triggers the release of dopamine in the brain, which leads to cravings and overeating. When you stop eating sugar, you are killing off the sugar parasites in your gut. These parasites are the ones hijacking your brain and sending messages for more sugar.

Finally, training yourself to crave fats is absolutely obtainable! This 28 day challenge is designed to make it as easy as possible. I am on like day 900 of this lifestyle and I am only asking you for 28.

MEAT DOES NOT CAUSE CANCER

DOCTORS ARE NOT HEALTH EXPERTS

WHAT YOU NEED

- 3 Days Off
- Low Stress
- Desire for Change

WHAT TO BUY

- MCT Oil
- Grass Fed Butter
- Electrolytes (I use LMNT)
- Nutritional Yeast or B12 Complex
- A Good Probiotic with over 25 billion cfu
  and at least 10 strains

IT IS TIME

You're about to embark on a journey that will transform not only your physical health, but your mental and emotional wellbeing as well. This 28-day health challenge is your opportunity to push yourself to new heights and reach your full potential. You're capable of achieving anything you set your mind to, and this challenge will test your limits, but the rewards will be worth it. As you begin this challenge, remember that every day is a chance to make progress towards your goals, and every small step forward is a victory. So get ready to crush your fears, overcome your obstacles, and emerge stronger, healthier, and happier than ever before.

Feel free to eat anything on the menu during each meal. In this book you will find over 100 amazing recipes and on top of that I included over 200 restaurants and exactly what to order at each one! In the beginning, you will feel like you do not have enough variety, but before you know it, you will be looking forward to eating pretty much the same thing everyday. The next 28 pages will outline your every move and make it as easy as possible! Hang in there and push through! It is time to optimize your life, reverse disease, lose weight, and live your happiest life.

THE OPTIMUM 28

DAY 1

TIME	TASK
WAKE UP	COFFEE OR TEA WITH 1 TSP MCT OIL AND 1 TSP GRASS FED BUTTER
9:00 - 10:00 AM	SIMPLE WORK OUT GO AS LONG AS YOU CAN WITHOUT EATING
10:00-12:00 PM	FIRST MEAL THE OPTIMUM BREAKFAST (121) BLACK AND WHITE FAT BOMB (127) HANDFUL OF NUTS EAT ALL YOU WANT 10 MINUTE WALK
12:00 - 1:00 PM	VITAMIN B12 COMPLEX ELECTROLYTES PROBIOTICS
1:00 - 4:00 PM	NO LUNCH! COFFEE OR TEA WITH MCT OIL AND OR BUTTER
6:00 - 8:00 PM	SECOND MEAL RIBEYE ASPARAGUS ARUGULA (109) BLACK AND WHITE FAT BOMB (127) HANDFUL OF NUTS EAT ALL YOU WANT
10:00 - BED	NO SNACKING! GO TO BED HUNGRY

IF YOU WERE REALLY HUNGRY DURING THE DAY, THEN MAKE SURE YOU EAT MORE FAT DURING YOUR FIRST MEAL. ADD BUTTER AND OLIVE OIL VERY LIBERALLY AND EAT MORE FAT BOMBS AND NUTS! GO BIG! ALSO DRINK A GLASS OF SALT WATER WHEN HUNGRY.

THE OPTIMUM 28

DAY 2

TIME	TASK
WAKE UP	COFFEE OR TEA WITH 1 TSP MCT OIL AND 1 TSP GRASS FED BUTTER
9:00 - 10:00 AM	SIMPLE WORK OUT GO AS LONG AS YOU CAN WITHOUT EATING!
10:00-12:00 PM	FIRST MEAL OPTIMUM BREAKFAST BOWL (99) CHOCOLATE AVOCADO MOUSSE (128) or HANDFUL OF NUTS EAT ALL YOU WANT! 10 MINUTE WALK
12:00 - 1:00 PM	VITAMIN B12 COMPLEX ELECTROLYTES PROBIOTICS
1:00 - 4:00 PM	NO LUNCH! NO SNACKS! (Have a coffee or tea with butter and MCT oil if you need)
6:00 - 8:00 PM	SECOND MEAL GRILLED CHICKEN ROASTED ASPARAGUS MUSHROOMS (81) CHOCOLATE AVOCADO MOUSSE (128) EAT ALL YOU WANT!
10:00 - BED	NO SNACKING! GO TO BED HUNGRY

THESE FIRST 3 DAYS ARE THE MOST DIFFICULT. YOU CAN DO IT! HANG IN THERE WHILE YOUR BODY ADAPTS TO USING FAT AS A RESOURCE.

THE OPTIMUM 28

DAY 3

TIME	TASK
WAKE UP	COFFEE OR TEA WITH 1 TSP MCT OIL AND 1 TSP GRASS FED BUTTER
9:00 - 10:00 AM	SIMPLE WORK OUT GO AS LONG AS YOU CAN WITHOUT EATING!
10:00-12:00 PM	FIRST MEAL SAUSAGE AND EGGS WITH HAMBURGER (112) FUDGY BROWNIES (129) EAT ALL YOU WANT! 10 MINUTE WALK
12:00 - 1:00 PM	VITAMIN B12 COMPLEX ELECTROLYTES PROBIOTICS
1:00 - 4:00 PM	NO LUNCH! NO SNACKS! (Have a coffee or tea with butter and MCT oil if you need)
6:00 - 8:00 PM	SECOND MEAL MEATLOAF MASHED GREEN BEANS (95) FUDGY BROWNIES (129) EAT ALL YOU WANT!
10:00 - BED	NO SNACKING! GO TO BED HUNGRY

THE OPTIMUM 28

DAY 4

TIME	TASK
WAKE UP	COFFEE OR TEA WITH 1 TSP MCT OIL AND 1 TSP GRASS FED BUTTER
9:00 - 10:00 AM	SIMPLE WORK OUT GO AS LONG AS YOU CAN WITHOUT EATING
10:00-12:00 PM	FIRST MEAL BACON CHEESEBURGER BREAKFAST BOWL (44) KETO CHEESECAKE (130) EAT ALL YOU WANT! 10 MINUTE WALK
12:00 - 1:00 PM	VITAMIN B12 COMPLEX ELECTROLYTES PROBIOTICS
1:00 - 4:00 PM	NO LUNCH! NO SNACKS! (Have a coffee or tea with butter and MCT oil if you need)
6:00 - 8:00 PM	SECOND MEAL BAKED SALMON WITH DILL AND BROCCOLI (50) KETO CHEESECAKE (130) HANDFUL OF NUTS EAT ALL YOU WANT!
10:00 - BED	NO SNACKING! GO TO BED HUNGRY

THE OPTIMUM 28

DAY 5

TIME	TASK
WAKE UP	COFFEE OR TEA WITH 1 TSP MCT OIL AND 1 TSP GRASS FED BUTTER
9:00 - 10:00 AM	SIMPLE WORK OUT GO AS LONG AS YOU CAN WITHOUT EATING
10:00-12:00 PM	FIRST MEAL BAKED EGGS FLORENTINE (85) KETO CHOCOLATE ICE CREAM (131) EAT ALL YOU WANT! 10 MINUTE WALK
12:00 - 1:00 PM	VITAMIN B12 COMPLEX ELECTROLYTES PROBIOTICS
1:00 - 4:00 PM	NO LUNCH! NO SNACKS! (Have a coffee or tea with butter and MCT oil if you need)
6:00 - 8:00 PM	SECOND MEAL PORK CHOPS WITH ROASTED ASPARAGUS (104) KETO CHOCOLATE ICE CREAM (131) HANDFUL OF NUTS EAT ALL YOU WANT!
10:00 - BED	NO SNACKING! GO TO BED HUNGRY

THE OPTIMUM 28

DAY 6

TIME	TASK
WAKE UP	COFFEE OR TEA WITH 1 TSP MCT OIL AND 1 TSP GRASS FED BUTTER
9:00 - 10:00 AM	SIMPLE WORK OUT GO AS LONG AS YOU CAN WITHOUT EATING
10:00-12:00 PM	FIRST MEAL BAKED EGGS IN AVOCADO CUPS (49) COCONUT ALMOND FAT BOMBS (132) EAT ALL YOU WANT! 10 MINUTE WALK
12:00 - 1:00 PM	VITAMIN B12 COMPLEX ELECTROLYTES PROBIOTICS
1:00 - 4:00 PM	NO LUNCH! NO SNACKS! (Have a coffee or tea with butter and MCT oil if you need)
6:00 - 8:00 PM	SECOND MEAL BRAISED SHORT RIBS WITH CAULIFLOWER MASHED (63) COCONUT ALMOND FAT BOMBS (132) EAT ALL YOU WANT!
10:00 - BED	NO SNACKING! GO TO BED HUNGRY

THE OPTIMUM 28

DAY 7

TIME	TASK
WAKE UP	COFFEE OR TEA WITH 1 TSP MCT OIL AND 1 TSP GRASS FED BUTTER
9:00 - 10:00 AM	SIMPLE WORK OUT GO AS LONG AS YOU CAN WITHOUT EATING
10:00–12:00 PM	FIRST MEAL MEAT LOVERS OMELET WITH AVOCADO (94) LEMON CHEESECAKE (133) EAT ALL YOU WANT! 10 MINUTE WALK
12:00 - 1:00 PM	VITAMIN B12 COMPLEX ELECTROLYTES PROBIOTICS
1:00 - 4:00 PM	NO LUNCH! NO SNACKS! (Have a coffee or tea with butter and MCT oil if you need)
6:00 - 8:00 PM	SECOND MEAL NEW YORK STEAK WITH BACON WRAPPED GREEN BEANS (97) LEMON CHEESECAKE (133) EAT ALL YOU WANT!
10:00 - BED	NO SNACKING! GO TO BED HUNGRY

THE OPTIMUM 28

DAY 8

TIME	TASK
WAKE UP	COFFEE OR TEA WITH 1 TSP MCT OIL AND 1 TSP GRASS FED BUTTER
9:00 - 10:00 AM	SIMPLE WORK OUT GO AS LONG AS YOU CAN WITHOUT EATING
10:00-12:00 PM	FIRST MEAL PANCAKES AND SAUSAGE WITH BACON (102) MACAROONS (134) EAT ALL YOU WANT! 10 MINUTE WALK
12:00 - 1:00 PM	VITAMIN B12 COMPLEX ELECTROLYTES PROBIOTICS
1:00 - 4:00 PM	NO LUNCH! NO SNACKS! (Have a coffee or tea with butter and MCT oil if you need)
6:00 - 8:00 PM	SECOND MEAL BEEF PATTY AND CHICKEN FAJITAS (57) MACAROONS (134) HANDFUL OF NUTS EAT ALL YOU WANT!
10:00 - BED	NO SNACKING! GO TO BED HUNGRY

THE OPTIMUM 28

DAY 9

TIME	TASK
WAKE UP	COFFEE OR TEA WITH 1 TSP MCT OIL AND 1 TSP GRASS FED BUTTER
9:00 - 10:00 AM	SIMPLE WORK OUT GO AS LONG AS YOU CAN WITHOUT EATING
10:00-12:00 PM	FIRST MEAL MEAT LOVERS FRITTATA (93) MINT CHIP SMOOTHIE (135) EAT ALL YOU WANT! 10 MINUTE WALK
12:00 - 1:00 PM	VITAMIN B12 COMPLEX ELECTROLYTES PROBIOTICS
1:00 - 4:00 PM	NO LUNCH! NO SNACKS! (Have a coffee or tea with butter and MCT oil if you need)
6:00 - 8:00 PM	SECOND MEAL COBB SALAD WITH HAMBURGER PATTY (74) MINT CHIP SMOOTHIE (135) EAT ALL YOU WANT!
10:00 - BED	NO SNACKING! GO TO BED HUNGRY

THE OPTIMUM 28

DAY 10

TIME	TASK
WAKE UP	COFFEE OR TEA WITH 1 TSP MCT OIL AND 1 TSP GRASS FED BUTTER
9:00 - 10:00 AM	SIMPLE WORK OUT GO AS LONG AS YOU CAN WITHOUT EATING
10:00-12:00 PM	FIRST MEAL SAUSAGE PATTY SANDWICHES (113) PUMPKIN PIE (136) EAT ALL YOU WANT! 10 MINUTE WALK
12:00 - 1:00 PM	VITAMIN B12 COMPLEX ELECTROLYTES PROBIOTICS
1:00 - 4:00 PM	NO LUNCH! NO SNACKS! (Have a coffee or tea with butter and MCT oil if you need)
6:00 - 8:00 PM	SECOND MEAL FETA STUFFED CHICKEN BREAST WITH CAULIFLOWER MASHED (78) PUMPKIN PIE (136) EAT ALL YOU WANT!
10:00 - BED	NO SNACKING! GO TO BED HUNGRY

THE OPTIMUM 28

DAY II

TIME	TASK
WAKE UP	COFFEE OR TEA WITH 1 TSP MCT OIL AND 1 TSP GRASS FED BUTTER
9:00 - 10:00 AM	SIMPLE WORK OUT GO AS LONG AS YOU CAN WITHOUT EATING
10:00–12:00 PM	FIRST MEAL TURKEY PATTY WITH EGGS, BACON, AND AVOCADO (125) BLACK AND WHITE FAT BOMBS (127) EAT ALL YOU WANT! 10 MINUTE WALK
12:00 - 1:00 PM	VITAMIN B12 COMPLEX ELECTROLYTES PROBIOTICS
1:00 - 4:00 PM	NO LUNCH! NO SNACKS! (Have a coffee or tea with butter and MCT oil if you need)
6:00 - 8:00 PM	SECOND MEAL BUFFALO CHICKEN LETTUCE WRAPS (66) BLACK AND WHITE FAT BOMBS (127) HANDFUL OF NUTS EAT ALL YOU WANT!
10:00 - BED	NO SNACKING! GO TO BED HUNGRY

THE OPTIMUM 28

DAY 12

TIME	TASK
WAKE UP	COFFEE OR TEA WITH 1 TSP MCT OIL AND 1 TSP GRASS FED BUTTER
9:00 - 10:00 AM	SIMPLE WORK OUT GO AS LONG AS YOU CAN WITHOUT EATING
10:00-12:00 PM	FIRST MEAL NEW YORK STEAK AND EGGS WITH BACON (96) CHOCOLATE AVOCADO MOUSSE (128) EAT ALL YOU WANT! 10 MINUTE WALK
12:00 - 1:00 PM	VITAMIN B12 COMPLEX ELECTROLYTES PROBIOTICS
1:00 - 4:00 PM	NO LUNCH! NO SNACKS! (Have a coffee or tea with butter and MCT oil if you need)
6:00 - 8:00 PM	SECOND MEAL COCONUT CURRY CHICKEN WITH CAULIFLOWER RICE (75) CHOCOLATE AVOCADO MOUSSE (128) EAT ALL YOU WANT!
10:00 - BED	NO SNACKING! GO TO BED HUNGRY

THE OPTIMUM 28

DAY 13

TIME	TASK
WAKE UP	COFFEE OR TEA WITH 1 TSP MCT OIL AND 1 TSP GRASS FED BUTTER
9:00 - 10:00 AM	SIMPLE WORK OUT GO AS LONG AS YOU CAN WITHOUT EATING
10:00-12:00 PM	FIRST MEAL BREAKFAST CASSEROLE (87) FUDGY BROWNIES (129) EAT ALL YOU WANT! 10 MINUTE WALK
12:00 - 1:00 PM	VITAMIN B12 COMPLEX ELECTROLYTES PROBIOTICS
1:00 - 4:00 PM	NO LUNCH! NO SNACKS! (Have a coffee or tea with butter and MCT oil if you need)
6:00 - 8:00 PM	SECOND MEAL BEEF RIBS WITH ROASTED BROCCOLI (58) FUDGY BROWNIES (129) EAT ALL YOU WANT!
10:00 - BED	NO SNACKING! GO TO BED HUNGRY

THE OPTIMUM 28

DAY 14

TIME	TASK
WAKE UP	COFFEE OR TEA WITH 1 TSP MCT OIL AND 1 TSP GRASS FED BUTTER
9:00 - 10:00 AM	SIMPLE WORK OUT GO AS LONG AS YOU CAN WITHOUT EATING
10:00-12:00 PM	FIRST MEAL PORK CHOPS WITH EGGS (106) CHEESECAKE (130) EAT ALL YOU WANT! 10 MINUTE WALK
12:00 - 1:00 PM	VITAMIN B12 COMPLEX ELECTROLYTES PROBIOTICS
1:00 - 4:00 PM	NO LUNCH! NO SNACKS! (Have a coffee or tea with butter and MCT oil if you need)
6:00 - 8:00 PM	SECOND MEAL BACON WRAPPED SCALLOPS WITH BEEF PATTY (45) CHEESECAKE (130) EAT ALL YOU WANT!
10:00 - BED	NO SNACKING! GO TO BED HUNGRY

THE OPTIMUM 28

DAY 15

TIME	TASK
WAKE UP	COFFEE OR TEA WITH 1 TSP MCT OIL AND 1 TSP GRASS FED BUTTER
9:00 - 10:00 AM	SIMPLE WORK OUT GO AS LONG AS YOU CAN WITHOUT EATING
10:00-12:00 PM	FIRST MEAL OPTIMUM BEEF SCRAMBLE (98) 10 MINUTE WALK
12:00 - 1:00 PM	VITAMIN B12 COMPLEX ELECTROLYTES PROBIOTICS
1:00 - 4:00 PM	NO LUNCH! NO SNACKS!
6:00 - 8:00 PM	SECOND MEAL LAMB CHOPS WITH ROASTED ASPARAGUS (89)
10:00 - BED	NO SNACKING! GO TO BED HUNGRY

THE OPTIMUM 28

DAY 16

TIME	TASK
WAKE UP	COFFEE OR TEA WITH 1 TSP MCT OIL AND 1 TSP GRASS FED BUTTER
9:00 - 10:00 AM	SIMPLE WORK OUT GO AS LONG AS YOU CAN WITHOUT EATING
10:00-12:00 PM	FIRST MEAL BEEF LIVER WITH EGGS, BACON, AND ONION (55) 10 MINUTE WALK
12:00 - 1:00 PM	VITAMIN B12 COMPLEX ELECTROLYTES PROBIOTICS
1:00 - 4:00 PM	NO LUNCH! NO SNACKS!
6:00 - 8:00 PM	SECOND MEAL LETTUCE WRAPPED CHEESEBURGERS (92)
10:00 - BED	NO SNACKING! GO TO BED HUNGRY

THE OPTIMUM 28

DAY 17

TIME	TASK
WAKE UP	COFFEE OR TEA WITH 1 TSP MCT OIL AND 1 TSP GRASS FED BUTTER
9:00 - 10:00 AM	SIMPLE WORK OUT GO AS LONG AS YOU CAN WITHOUT EATING
10:00-12:00 PM	FIRST MEAL BEEFY EGGS AND AVOCADO (61) 10 MINUTE WALK
12:00 - 1:00 PM	VITAMIN B12 COMPLEX ELECTROLYTES PROBIOTICS
1:00 - 4:00 PM	NO LUNCH! NO SNACKS!
6:00 - 8:00 PM	SECOND MEAL TURKEY BURGER WITH ARUGULA (123)
10:00 - BED	NO SNACKING! GO TO BED HUNGRY

THE OPTIMUM 28
DAY 18

TIME	TASK
WAKE UP	COFFEE OR TEA WITH 1 TSP MCT OIL AND 1 TSP GRASS FED BUTTER
9:00 - 10:00 AM	SIMPLE WORK OUT GO AS LONG AS YOU CAN WITHOUT EATING
10:00-12:00 PM	FIRST MEAL MEAT LOVERS OMELET WITH AVOCADO (94) 10 MINUTE WALK
12:00 - 1:00 PM	VITAMIN B12 COMPLEX ELECTROLYTES PROBIOTICS
1:00 - 4:00 PM	NO LUNCH! NO SNACKS!
6:00 - 8:00 PM	SECOND MEAL RIBEYE ASPARAGUS WITH ARUGULA (109)
10:00 - BED	NO SNACKING! GO TO BED HUNGRY

THE OPTIMUM 28

DAY 19

TIME	TASK
WAKE UP	COFFEE OR TEA WITH 1 TSP MCT OIL AND 1 TSP GRASS FED BUTTER
9:00 - 10:00 AM	SIMPLE WORK OUT GO AS LONG AS YOU CAN WITHOUT EATING
10:00-12:00 PM	FIRST MEAL POACHED EGGS WITH SAUSAGE (105) 10 MINUTE WALK
12:00 - 1:00 PM	VITAMIN B12 COMPLEX ELECTROLYTES PROBIOTICS
1:00 - 4:00 PM	NO LUNCH! NO SNACKS!
6:00 - 8:00 PM	SECOND MEAL STEAK SALAD WITH AVOCADO (118)
10:00 - BED	NO SNACKING! GO TO BED HUNGRY

THE OPTIMUM 28

DAY 20

TIME	TASK
WAKE UP	COFFEE OR TEA WITH 1 TSP MCT OIL AND 1 TSP GRASS FED BUTTER
9:00 - 10:00 AM	SIMPLE WORK OUT GO AS LONG AS YOU CAN WITHOUT EATING
10:00-12:00 PM	FIRST MEAL SPINACH AND MUSHROOM OMELET WITH BURGER PATTY (117) 10 MINUTE WALK
12:00 - 1:00 PM	VITAMIN B12 COMPLEX ELECTROLYTES PROBIOTICS
1:00 - 4:00 PM	NO LUNCH! NO SNACKS!
6:00 - 8:00 PM	SECOND MEAL TURKEY MEATLOAF WITH GREEN BEANS (124)
10:00 - BED	NO SNACKING! GO TO BED HUNGRY

THE OPTIMUM 28

DAY 21

TIME	TASK
WAKE UP	COFFEE OR TEA WITH 1 TSP MCT OIL AND 1 TSP GRASS FED BUTTER
9:00 - 10:00 AM	SIMPLE WORK OUT GO AS LONG AS YOU CAN WITHOUT EATING
10:00-12:00 PM	FIRST MEAL GARLIC STEAK BITES WITH EGGS AND BACON (80) 10 MINUTE WALK
12:00 - 1:00 PM	VITAMIN B12 COMPLEX ELECTROLYTES PROBIOTICS
1:00 - 4:00 PM	NO LUNCH! NO SNACKS!
6:00 - 8:00 PM	SECOND MEAL BUFFALO CHICKEN SALAD WITH BLUE CHEESE (67)
10:00 - BED	NO SNACKING! GO TO BED HUNGRY

THE OPTIMUM 28

DAY 22

TIME	TASK
WAKE UP	COFFEE OR TEA WITH 1 TSP MCT OIL AND 1 TSP GRASS FED BUTTER
9:00 - 10:00 AM	SIMPLE WORK OUT GO AS LONG AS YOU CAN WITHOUT EATING
10:00-12:00 PM	FIRST MEAL BACON EGGS AND A BEEF PATTY (46) 10 MINUTE WALK
12:00 - 1:00 PM	VITAMIN B12 COMPLEX ELECTROLYTES PROBIOTICS
1:00 - 4:00 PM	NO LUNCH! NO SNACKS!
6:00 - 8:00 PM	SECOND MEAL BEEF TACOS IN LETTUCE WRAPS (60)
10:00 - BED	NO SNACKING! GO TO BED HUNGRY

THE OPTIMUM 28

DAY 23

TIME	TASK
WAKE UP	COFFEE OR TEA WITH 1 TSP MCT OIL AND 1 TSP GRASS FED BUTTER
9:00 - 10:00 AM	SIMPLE WORK OUT GO AS LONG AS YOU CAN WITHOUT EATING
10:00-12:00 PM	FIRST MEAL SAUSAGE PATTY SANDWICHES (113) 10 MINUTE WALK
12:00 - 1:00 PM	VITAMIN B12 COMPLEX ELECTROLYTES PROBIOTICS
1:00 - 4:00 PM	NO LUNCH! NO SNACKS!
6:00 - 8:00 PM	SECOND MEAL SHRIMP AND BURGER PATTY WITH ASPARAGUS (115)
10:00 - BED	NO SNACKING! GO TO BED HUNGRY

THE OPTIMUM 28

DAY 24

TIME	TASK
WAKE UP	COFFEE OR TEA WITH 1 TSP MCT OIL AND 1 TSP GRASS FED BUTTER
9:00 - 10:00 AM	SIMPLE WORK OUT GO AS LONG AS YOU CAN WITHOUT EATING
10:00-12:00 PM	FIRST MEAL OPTIMUM BREAKFAST BOWL (99) 10 MINUTE WALK
12:00 - 1:00 PM	VITAMIN B12 COMPLEX ELECTROLYTES PROBIOTICS
1:00 - 4:00 PM	NO LUNCH! NO SNACKS!
6:00 - 8:00 PM	SECOND MEAL TOMATO SOUP WITH GRILLED CHEESE BITES (122)
10:00 - BED	NO SNACKING! GO TO BED HUNGRY

THE OPTIMUM 28

DAY 25

TIME	TASK
WAKE UP	COFFEE OR TEA WITH 1 TSP MCT OIL AND 1 TSP GRASS FED BUTTER
9:00 - 10:00 AM	SIMPLE WORK OUT GO AS LONG AS YOU CAN WITHOUT EATING
10:00-12:00 PM	FIRST MEAL THE OPTIMUM BEEF SCRAMBLE (98) 10 MINUTE WALK
12:00 - 1:00 PM	VITAMIN B12 COMPLEX ELECTROLYTES PROBIOTICS
1:00 - 4:00 PM	NO LUNCH! NO SNACKS!
6:00 - 8:00 PM	SECOND MEAL RIBEYE WITH CREAMED SPINACH AND MUSHROOMS (111)
10:00 - BED	NO SNACKING! GO TO BED HUNGRY

THE OPTIMUM 28

DAY 26

TIME	TASK
WAKE UP	COFFEE OR TEA WITH 1 TSP MCT OIL AND 1 TSP GRASS FED BUTTER
9:00 - 10:00 AM	SIMPLE WORK OUT GO AS LONG AS YOU CAN WITHOUT EATING
10:00-12:00 PM	FIRST MEAL PORK CHOPS WITH EGGS, AVOCADO (106) 10 MINUTE WALK
12:00 - 1:00 PM	VITAMIN B12 COMPLEX ELECTROLYTES PROBIOTICS
1:00 - 4:00 PM	NO LUNCH! NO SNACKS!
6:00 - 8:00 PM	SECOND MEAL STEAK SALAD WITH AVOCADO (118)
10:00 - BED	NO SNACKING! GO TO BED HUNGRY

THE OPTIMUM 28

DAY 27

TIME	TASK
WAKE UP	COFFEE OR TEA WITH 1 TSP MCT OIL AND 1 TSP GRASS FED BUTTER
9:00 - 10:00 AM	SIMPLE WORK OUT GO AS LONG AS YOU CAN WITHOUT EATING
10:00-12:00 PM	FIRST MEAL GARLIC STEAK BITES WITH EGGS AND BACON (80) 10 MINUTE WALK
12:00 - 1:00 PM	VITAMIN B12 COMPLEX ELECTROLYTES PROBIOTICS
1:00 - 4:00 PM	NO LUNCH! NO SNACKS!
6:00 - 8:00 PM	SECOND MEAL EGGPLANT PARMESAN (77)
10:00 - BED	NO SNACKING! GO TO BED HUNGRY

THE OPTIMUM 28

DAY 28

TIME	TASK
WAKE UP	COFFEE OR TEA WITH 1 TSP MCT OIL AND 1 TSP GRASS FED BUTTER
9:00 - 10:00 AM	SIMPLE WORK OUT GO AS LONG AS YOU CAN WITHOUT EATING
10:00-12:00 PM	FIRST MEAL BAKED EGGS FLORENTINE (85) 10 MINUTE WALK
12:00 - 1:00 PM	VITAMIN B12 COMPLEX ELECTROLYTES PROBIOTICS
1:00 - 4:00 PM	NO LUNCH! NO SNACKS!
6:00 - 8:00 PM	SECOND MEAL BEEF BRISKET WITH GREEN BEANS (53)
10:00 - BED	NO SNACKING! GO TO BED HUNGRY

ALMOND-CRUSTED BACON and TOMATO QUICHE

What You Need

- 1 cup almond flour
- 1/4 cup melted butter
- 1/4 teaspoon salt
- 6 slices of bacon, cooked and crumbled
- 1/2 cup cherry tomatoes, halved
- 1/2 cup shredded cheese
- 4 large eggs
- 1/2 cup heavy cream
- 1/2 teaspoon salt
- 1/4 teaspoon black pepper

How To Cook

- Preheat your oven to 350°F (175°C) and grease a 9-inch pie or tart pan.
- In a medium bowl, mix together the almond flour, melted butter, and salt until well combined.
- Press the almond flour mixture evenly onto the bottom and up the sides of the prepared pan to form the crust.
- Bake the crust in the preheated oven for 8-10 minutes, or until lightly golden brown. Remove from the oven and set aside.
- In a large bowl, whisk together the eggs, heavy cream, salt, and black pepper until well combined.
- Stir in the crumbled bacon, halved cherry tomatoes, shredded cheese into the egg mixture.
- Pour the egg and filling mixture into the almond crust in the pan.
- Bake the quiche in the preheated oven for 25-30 minutes, or until the center is set and the top is lightly golden brown.
- Remove, let sit for 5 and then enjoy!

BABY BACK RIBS and BRUSSEL SPROUTS with LEMON

What You Need

- 1/2 rack of baby back ribs
- 1/2 cup melted butter
- 2 tbsp coconut oil
- 1 tbsp paprika
- 1 tbsp garlic powder
- 1 tbsp onion powder
- 1 tbsp dried thyme
- 1 tbsp dried rosemary
- 1/2 tbsp salt
- 1/2 tbsp black pepper
- 1/2 cup Brussels sprouts, trimmed and halved
- 2 tbsp butter
- 1 tbsp fresh lemon juice
- 1 tsp lemon zest

How To Cook

- Preheat your oven to 300°F (150°C).
- Prepare the baby back ribs by removing the membrane from the back of the ribs. In a bowl, mix together melted butter, coconut oil, paprika, garlic powder, onion powder, thyme, rosemary, salt, and black pepper to make a marinade.
- Coat the half rack of ribs with the marinade, making sure to cover it evenly on both sides. Place the ribs on a baking sheet lined with foil, bone side down.
- Bake the ribs in the preheated oven for 2 to 2 1/2 hours, until they are tender and cooked through.
- While the ribs are cooking, prepare the Brussels sprouts. In a small skillet over medium-high heat, melt the butter. Add the halved Brussels sprouts and cook, stirring occasionally, until they are browned and crispy, about 10 minutes. Season with salt and pepper to taste. Set aside.
- For the lemon sauce, whisk together melted butter, fresh lemon juice, salt, pepper, lemon zest. Enjoy!

BACON CHEESEBURGER BOWL

What You Need

- 2 large eggs
- 4 slices of bacon
- 1/2 cup shredded cheese (such as cheddar or Monterey Jack)
- 1 small avocado, diced
- 2 tablespoons grass-fed butter
- 2 tablespoons olive oil
- 1 tablespoon nutritional yeast
- Salt and pepper to taste

How To Cook

- Cook the bacon in a skillet over medium heat until crispy. Once cooked, transfer the bacon to a paper towel-lined plate to drain excess grease. Crumble the bacon into small pieces.
- In the same skillet, add 1 tablespoon of grass-fed butter and melt over medium heat. Crack the eggs into the skillet and cook until the whites are set but the yolks are still slightly runny, or to your desired level of doneness. Season the eggs with salt and pepper to taste.
- In a separate small bowl, toss the diced avocado with 1 tablespoon of olive oil, and season with a pinch of salt and pepper.
- In a medium bowl, combine the cooked bacon, shredded cheese, and seasoned avocado.
- Once the eggs are cooked, carefully transfer them on top of the bacon, cheese, and avocado mixture in the bowl.
- Melt the remaining 1 tablespoon of grass-fed butter in the skillet, then drizzle it over the eggs and the rest of the ingredients in the bowl.
- Sprinkle the nutritional yeast over the top of the bowl.
- Finish by drizzling the remaining 1 tablespoon of olive oil over the top of the bowl.

BACON WRAPPED SCALLOPS with BEEF PATTY

What You Need

- 12 large scallops
- 12 slices of bacon
- Salt and pepper to taste
- 1/2 lb ground beef
- 1/2 teaspoon garlic powder
- 1/2 teaspoon onion powder
- 1/2 teaspoon salt
- 1/4 teaspoon black pepper
- 1 tablespoon cooking oil or butter
- 2 cups broccoli florets

How To Cook

- Preheat your oven to 375°F (190°C).
- Wrap each scallop with a slice of bacon and secure with a toothpick. Season with a little salt and pepper.
- In a separate bowl, mix together the ground beef, garlic powder, onion powder, salt, and black pepper. Form the mixture into 2 beef patties.
- Heat a skillet over medium-high heat and add cooking oil or butter.
- Add the beef patties to the skillet and cook for about 3-4 minutes per side, or until they are cooked to your desired level of doneness. Transfer the beef patties to a baking sheet.
- Place the bacon-wrapped scallops on the same baking sheet with the beef patties.
- Bake in the preheated oven for 12-15 minutes, or until the scallops are cooked and the bacon is crispy.
- While the scallops and beef patties are baking, steam or sauté the broccoli florets until they are tender.
- Once the scallops, beef patties, and broccoli are cooked, remove them from the oven and skillet, respectively.
- Serve hot, and enjoy your high-fat keto bacon-wrapped scallops with beef patty and broccoli!

BACON EGGS and a BEEF PATTY

What You Need

- 2 slices of bacon
- 1 beef patty
- 2 large eggs
- Salt and pepper to taste
- Optional toppings: sliced avocado, sliced tomato, shredded cheese

How To Cook

- Preheat a skillet over medium heat.
- Cook the bacon in the skillet until crispy, about 5-7 minutes, then remove from the skillet and place on a paper towel to drain excess grease.
- In the same skillet, cook the beef patty to your desired level of doneness, about 3-4 minutes per side for medium.
- Once the beef patty is cooked, remove it from the skillet and place on a plate.
- Crack the eggs into the same skillet and cook to your desired level of doneness. For sunny-side-up eggs, cook for about 3 minutes until the egg whites are set but the yolks are still runny.
- Once the eggs are cooked, remove them from the skillet and place on the same plate as the beef patty.
- Place the bacon on the plate with the beef patty and eggs.
- Season the eggs and beef patty with salt and pepper to taste, and top with any desired toppings.
- Enjoy your simple and delicious meal with bacon, eggs, and a beef patty!

BAKED CHICKEN THIGHS and BROCCOLI

What You Need

- 2 chicken thighs, bone-in and skin-on
- Broccoli florets
- Grass-fed butter
- Salt
- Olive oil

How To Cook

- Preheat your oven to 400°F (200°C).
- Place the chicken thighs on a baking sheet lined with parchment paper. Pat them dry with a paper towel to remove any excess moisture. Rub the chicken thighs generously with grass-fed butter on all sides, and sprinkle them with salt to taste.
- Toss the broccoli florets in olive oil and sprinkle with salt to taste.
- Place the seasoned chicken thighs and broccoli florets in the preheated oven. Roast for 25-30 minutes, or until the internal temperature of the chicken thighs reaches 165°F (74°C) and the broccoli is tender and lightly browned.
- Remove the chicken thighs and broccoli from the oven and let them rest for a few minutes before serving.
- To serve, place a chicken thigh on a plate and surround it with roasted broccoli florets. Drizzle additional melted grass-fed butter over the chicken and broccoli for added flavor and richness.
- Enjoy your delicious meal with juicy chicken thighs and roasted broccoli, flavored with grass-fed butter and olive oil!

BAKED CHICKEN WINGS with CELERY

What You Need

For the Chicken Wings:

- 1 lb chicken wings
- 1/4 cup melted butter
- 2 tbsp avocado oil or coconut oil
- 1 tbsp paprika
- 1 tbsp garlic powder
- 1 tbsp onion powder
- 1 tsp salt
- 1/2 tsp black pepper

For the Blue Cheese Dip:

- 1/2 cup sour cream
- 1/4 cup avocado mayonnaise
- 1/4 cup crumbled blue cheese
- 1 tbsp fresh lemon juice
- 1/2 tsp garlic powder
- Salt and pepper to taste
- celery sticks

How To Cook

- Preheat your oven to 400°F (200°C) and line a baking sheet with foil.
- In a bowl, mix together melted butter, avocado oil or coconut oil, paprika, garlic powder, onion powder, salt, and black pepper to make a marinade.
- Pat dry the chicken wings with paper towels and place them in a large bowl. Pour the marinade over the chicken wings and toss to coat them evenly.
- Arrange the chicken wings on the lined baking sheet in a single layer, leaving some space between each wing. Bake in the preheated oven for 30-35 minutes, flipping the wings halfway through, until they are crispy and cooked through.
- While the chicken wings are baking, prepare the blue cheese dip. In a small bowl, whisk together sour cream, mayonnaise, crumbled blue cheese, lemon juice, garlic powder, salt, and pepper. Taste and adjust seasoning as desired.
- Plate and enjoy!

BAKED EGGS in AVOCADO CUPS with BACON and CHEDDAR CHEESE

What You Need

- 2 ripe avocados
- 4 large eggs
- 4 slices of bacon
- 1/2 cup shredded cheddar cheese
- 2 tablespoons grass-fed butter, melted
- 1 tablespoon nutritional yeast
- Salt and pepper, to taste
- Fresh parsley, for garnish (optional)

How To Cook

- Preheat your oven to 375°F (190°C) and line a baking sheet with parchment paper.
- Cut the avocados in half and remove the pits. Scoop out a small portion of the flesh from each half to create a larger cavity for the eggs. Reserve the scooped out avocado flesh for later use.
- Place the avocado halves on the prepared baking sheet, resting them securely on the skin side to prevent them from rolling.
- In a skillet over medium heat, cook the bacon slices until crispy. Remove from the skillet and place on paper towels to drain excess grease. Once cooled, crumble the bacon into small pieces.
- In a bowl, mix the melted grass-fed butter, nutritional yeast, salt, and pepper.
- Spoon a small amount of the butter mixture into each avocado cavity. Reserve the remaining mixture for later use.
- Crack an egg into each avocado half, making sure not to overflow the cavity.
- Sprinkle the shredded cheddar cheese and crumbled bacon over the eggs.
- Drizzle the remaining butter mixture over the top of the avocados.
- Bake in the preheated oven for 15-20 minutes, or until the egg whites are set but the yolks are still slightly runny.
- Remove from the oven and let the baked eggs in avocado cups cool for a few minutes.
- Garnish with fresh parsley, if desired. Enjoy!

BAKED SALMON with DILL and BROCCOLI

What You Need

- 1 salmon filet (about 6 ounces)
- 1 cup broccoli florets
- 1 tablespoon unsalted butter, melted
- 1 teaspoon fresh dill, minced
- 1 clove garlic, minced
- Salt and pepper, to taste
- Lemon wedge, for serving

How To Cook

- Preheat your oven to 400°F (200°C). Line a small baking sheet with foil or parchment paper for easy cleanup.
- Place the salmon filet on the prepared baking sheet. Arrange the broccoli florets around the salmon filet.
- In a small bowl, mix together the melted butter, minced dill, minced garlic, salt, and pepper.
- Brush the butter mixture generously over the salmon filet and broccoli florets, reserving a little bit for later.
- Bake in the preheated oven for 12-15 minutes, or until the salmon is cooked through and flakes easily with a fork, and the broccoli is tender and lightly browned.
- Remove from the oven and drizzle the remaining butter mixture over the top of the salmon and broccoli.
- Serve the keto baked salmon with dill and broccoli hot, with a lemon wedge for squeezing over the top for added freshness.
- Enjoy your delicious and healthy keto baked salmon with dill and broccoli, perfect for a satisfying single serving meal!

BEEF BONE BROTH

What You Need

- 4-5 lbs grass fed grass finished beef bones (marrow and knuckle bones work well)
- 2 tbsp apple cider vinegar
- 3-4 quarts water
- 2 medium onions, quartered
- 3-4 garlic cloves, peeled and smashed
- 2 celery stalks, chopped
- 2 medium carrots, chopped
- 1 tbsp black peppercorns
- 1 bay leaf
- 1 tbsp dried thyme

How To Cook

- Preheat your oven to 450°F.
- Place the beef bones on a baking sheet and roast them in the preheated oven for 30-45 minutes until they are browned and caramelized. This step is optional, but it will add depth of flavor to the broth.
- Place the roasted bones in a large stockpot or slow cooker.
- Add the apple cider vinegar and enough water to cover the bones by about 2 inches.
- Let the bones and water mixture sit for 30 minutes to an hour to allow the vinegar to help extract the nutrients from the bones.
- Add the onions, garlic, celery, carrots, black peppercorns, bay leaf, and dried thyme to the stockpot or slow cooker.
- Bring the mixture to a boil, then reduce the heat to low and let it simmer for 12-24 hours. The longer the broth simmers, the more flavorful and nutritious it will be.
- Skim any foam or impurities that rise to the surface during the cooking process.
- After simmering, let the broth cool slightly and strain it through a fine-mesh strainer or cheesecloth into a large bowl or pot.
- Discard the solids and let the broth cool completely.
- Enjoy!

BEEF BONE MARROW with PARSLEY and GARLIC

What You Need

- 4-6 beef bone marrow bones
- Salt and pepper, to taste
- 2 cloves garlic, minced
- 1/4 cup fresh parsley, chopped
- 2 tablespoons olive oil

How To Cook

- Place the beef bone marrow bones on a baking sheet lined with parchment paper or a silicone mat.
- Season the bones with salt and pepper to taste.
- Roast the bones in the oven for 15-20 minutes, or until the marrow is cooked through and bubbling.
- While the bones are roasting, prepare the parsley and garlic topping. In a small bowl, mix together the minced garlic, chopped parsley, and olive oil until well combined.

- Once the bones are cooked, remove them from the oven and let them cool for a few minutes.
- To serve, spoon some of the parsley and garlic topping onto each bone marrow bone.
- Enjoy your delicious and nutritious beef bone marrow with parsley and garlic as a tasty appetizer or snack!

BEEF BRISKET with GREEN BEANS

What You Need

For the beef brisket:

- 3-4 lb beef brisket
- 2 tablespoons olive oil
- 1 teaspoon garlic powder
- 1 teaspoon onion powder
- 1 teaspoon smoked paprika
- 1/2 teaspoon dried oregano
- 1/2 teaspoon dried thyme
- 1/2 teaspoon salt
- 1/4 teaspoon black pepper

For the green beans:

- 1 lb fresh green beans, trimmed
- 2 tablespoons butter
- 2 cloves garlic, minced
- Salt and pepper, to taste

How To Cook

- Preheat your oven to 325°F.
- In a small bowl, mix together the garlic powder, onion powder, smoked paprika, dried oregano, dried thyme, salt, and black pepper.
- Rub the spice mixture all over the beef brisket, making sure to coat it evenly.
- Heat the olive oil in a large oven-safe Dutch oven over medium-high heat. Add the beef brisket and sear it on all sides until browned, about 3-4 minutes per side.
- Cover the Dutch oven with a lid and transfer it to the preheated oven. Bake the beef brisket for 3-4 hours, or until it is tender and falls apart easily with a fork.
- While the beef brisket is cooking, prepare the green beans. Bring a large pot of salted water to a boil. Add the trimmed green beans and blanch them for 2-3 minutes, or until they are bright green and just tender.
- Drain the green beans and immediately transfer them to a bowl of ice water to stop the cooking process. Drain again and set aside.
- In a large skillet, melt the butter over medium heat. Add the minced garlic and sauté for 30 seconds, or until fragrant.
- Add the blanched green beans to the skillet and toss to coat them in the garlic butter. Enjoy!

BEEF BURGERS with BACON and CHEESE

What You Need

- 1 lb. ground beef
- 1 egg
- 1 tbsp. Worcestershire sauce
- 1 tbsp. Dijon mustard
- 1 tsp. garlic powder
- Salt and pepper, to taste
- 4 slices of bacon
- 4 slices of cheddar cheese

How To Cook

- Preheat the grill to medium-high heat.
- In a large bowl, mix together the ground beef, egg, Worcestershire sauce, Dijon mustard, garlic powder, salt, and pepper. Form the mixture into four patties.
- Place the patties on the grill and cook for 4-5 minutes on each side, or until they are cooked to your desired level of doneness.
- While the beef burgers are cooking, fry the bacon in a skillet until crispy.
- Once the beef burgers are cooked, place a slice of cheese on top of each patty and let it melt for 1-2 minutes.
- Place each beef burger on a plate and top with a slice of bacon.
- Serve hot and enjoy your delicious beef burgers with bacon and cheese!

BEEF LIVER with BACON and ONIONS

What You Need

- 1/2 lb beef liver, thinly sliced
- 4 large eggs
- 4 slices of bacon
- 1/2 medium onion, thinly sliced
- 1 tablespoon of nutritional yeast
- Salt and pepper to taste
- Cooking oil or butter for frying

How To Cook

- In a skillet, cook the bacon slices over medium heat until crispy. Remove the bacon from the skillet and set aside, leaving the bacon grease in the skillet.
- Add the thinly sliced beef liver to the skillet with the bacon grease and cook over medium heat until the liver is cooked through and no longer pink, about 2-3 minutes per side. Remove the beef liver from the skillet and set aside.
- In the same skillet, add a little cooking oil or butter if needed, and then add the thinly sliced onion. Cook the onion over medium heat until softened and caramelized, about 5-7 minutes.
- Crack the eggs into the skillet with the caramelized onion, and season with nutritional yeast and salt and pepper to taste. Cook the eggs to your desired level of doneness, either sunny-side up or over-easy.
- Once the eggs are cooked, transfer the beef liver slices back to the skillet with the eggs and onions, and briefly heat through.
- Serve the beef liver and eggs with bacon and onions hot, and crumble the crispy bacon on top for added flavor and crunch.

BEEF MEATBALLS with TOMATO SAUCE

What You Need

For the meatballs:

- 2 pounds ground beef
- 1/2 cup almond flour
- 2 eggs
- 1/4 cup grated Parmesan cheese
- 1/4 cup chopped fresh parsley
- 1 tablespoon minced garlic
- 1 teaspoon dried oregano
- 1/2 teaspoon salt
- 1/2 teaspoon black pepper

For the Tomato Sauce

- 1 tablespoon olive oil
- 1/2 cup chopped onion
- 2 cloves garlic, minced
- 1 can (28 ounces) crushed tomatoes
- 1 teaspoon dried oregano
- 1/2 teaspoon salt
- 1/4 teaspoon black pepper

How To Cook

- Preheat your oven to 375°F.
- In a large bowl, combine the ground beef, almond flour, eggs, grated Parmesan cheese, chopped fresh parsley, minced garlic, dried oregano, salt, and black pepper. Mix until well combined.
- Shape the beef mixture into 2-inch meatballs and place them on a baking sheet lined with parchment paper.
- Bake the meatballs in the preheated oven for 20-25 minutes, or until cooked through and lightly browned.
- While the meatballs are baking, prepare the tomato sauce. In a large saucepan, heat the olive oil over medium-high heat. Add the chopped onion and sauté for 3-4 minutes, or until softened.
- Add the minced garlic to the saucepan and sauté for 30 seconds, or until fragrant.
- Add the crushed tomatoes, dried oregano, salt, and black pepper to the saucepan and stir to combine. Bring the sauce to a simmer and let it cook for 10-15 minutes, or until thickened.
- Once the meatballs are cooked, remove them from the oven and transfer them to the saucepan with the tomato sauce. Gently stir to coat the meatballs in the sauce.
- Plate and enjoy!

BEEF PATTY and CHICKEN FAJITAS

What You Need

For the Chicken Fajitas:
- 1 lb chicken breasts or thighs, thinly sliced
- 1 red bell pepper, thinly sliced
- 1 green bell pepper, thinly sliced
- 1 small red onion, thinly sliced
- 2 cloves garlic, minced
- 2 tbsp olive oil or avocado oil
- 1 tbsp chili powder
- 1 tsp cumin
- 1/2 tsp paprika
- 1/4 tsp cayenne pepper (optional for extra spice)
- Salt and black pepper to taste

For the Beef Patty:
- 8 oz ground beef
- Salt and black pepper to taste
- Cooking oil or butter for frying

How To Cook

For the Chicken Fajitas:
- In a large bowl, combine the sliced chicken, bell peppers, onion, minced garlic, olive oil or avocado oil, chili powder, cumin, paprika, cayenne pepper (if using), salt, and black pepper. Toss to coat the chicken and vegetables in the spices.
- Heat a large skillet or a cast-iron skillet over medium-high heat. Add the chicken and vegetables to the skillet and cook for 5-7 minutes, stirring occasionally, until the chicken is cooked through and the vegetables are tender and slightly charred. Remove from the skillet and set aside.

For the Beef Patty:
- Season the ground beef with salt and black pepper to taste. Shape the beef into a patty.
- Heat a separate skillet over medium-high heat and add cooking oil or butter. Enjoy!

BEEF RIBS and ROASTED BROCCOLI

What You Need

For the beef ribs:

- 2 lbs. beef ribs
- 1 tbsp. paprika
- 1 tbsp. garlic powder
- 1 tbsp. onion powder
- 1 tsp. dried oregano
- 1 tsp. salt
- 1/2 tsp. black pepper
- 1 tbsp. olive oil

For the roasted broccoli:

- 1 head of broccoli, cut into florets
- 2 tbsp. olive oil
- Salt and pepper, to taste

How To Cook

- Preheat the oven to 350°F.
- In a small bowl, mix together the paprika, garlic powder, onion powder, oregano, salt, and black pepper.
- Rub the spice mixture all over the beef ribs, making sure to coat both sides.
- Heat a large skillet over medium-high heat. Once hot, add the olive oil.
- Add the beef ribs to the skillet and cook for 2-3 minutes on each side, or until they are browned on the outside.
- Transfer the beef ribs to a baking dish and cover with foil.
- Place the baking dish in the oven and bake for 2-3 hours, or until the beef ribs are tender and cooked through.
- While the beef ribs are cooking, prepare the roasted broccoli. Place the broccoli florets on a baking sheet and drizzle with olive oil. Season with salt and pepper.
- Place the baking sheet in the oven and roast the broccoli for 20-25 minutes, or until they are tender and lightly browned.
- Once the beef ribs and broccoli are done, serve them together on a plate. Enjoy!

BEEF STEW

What You Need

- 2 lbs beef chuck roast, cut into bite-sized pieces
- Salt and black pepper, to taste
- 2 tbsp olive oil or coconut oil
- 1 large onion, chopped
- 3 cloves garlic, minced
- 2 cups beef broth
- 1 cup diced tomatoes, canned or fresh
- 2 tbsp tomato paste
- 2 tsp paprika
- 1 tsp dried thyme
- 1/2 tsp dried rosemary
- 1/2 tsp dried oregano
- 1/2 tsp ground cumin
- 1/4 tsp cayenne pepper
- 2 medium carrots, chopped
- 2 stalks celery, chopped
- 1 medium turnip, chopped
- 1 small rutabaga, chopped
- 1 small zucchini, chopped

How To Cook

- Season the beef pieces with salt and black pepper.
- Heat the olive oil or coconut oil in a large pot or Dutch oven over medium-high heat.
- Add the beef pieces to the pot and cook for 5-7 minutes until browned on all sides. Remove the beef from the pot and set aside.
- In the same pot, add the chopped onion and cook for 2-3 minutes until softened.
- Add the minced garlic to the pot and cook for another minute until fragrant.
- Add the beef broth, diced tomatoes, tomato paste, paprika, thyme, rosemary, oregano, cumin, and cayenne pepper to the pot. Stir to combine.
- Add the chopped carrots, celery, turnip, and rutabaga to the pot. Stir to combine.
- Bring the mixture to a boil then reduce the heat to low and let it simmer for 45 minutes
- Add the chopped zucchini to the pot and let it cook for another 10-15 minutes until tender.

BEEF TACOS in LETTUCE WRAPS

What You Need

- 1 lb ground beef
- 1 tbsp olive oil
- 1/2 cup diced onion
- 2 cloves garlic, minced
- 1 tbsp chili powder
- 1 tsp ground cumin
- 1/2 tsp paprika
- 1/4 tsp cayenne pepper (optional)
- Salt and black pepper, to taste
- 1/2 cup diced tomatoes
- 2 tbsp chopped fresh cilantro
- 1 head of lettuce, such as butter lettuce or iceberg lettuce
- Toppings of your choice, such as shredded cheese, diced avocado, and sour cream

How To Cook

- Heat the olive oil in a large skillet over medium-high heat.
- Add the diced onion to the skillet and cook for 2-3 minutes until softened.
- Add the minced garlic to the skillet and cook for another minute until fragrant.
- Add the ground beef to the skillet and cook for 5-7 minutes until browned and cooked through, breaking it up with a wooden spoon as it cooks.
- Add the chili powder, ground cumin, paprika, cayenne pepper (if using), salt, and black pepper to the skillet. Stir to combine.
- Add the diced tomatoes to the skillet and cook for another 2-3 minutes until heated through.
- Remove the skillet from the heat and stir in the chopped fresh cilantro.
- Wash and dry the lettuce leaves and use them as taco shells to serve the beef mixture.
- Top the lettuce tacos with your desired toppings, such as shredded cheese, diced avocado, and sour cream. Enjoy

BEEFY EGGS and AVOCADO

What You Need

- 1/2 pound ground beef
- 1 tablespoon coconut oil
- 4 large eggs
- 1/2 avocado
- Salt and pepper, to taste

How To Cook

- Preheat a skillet over medium heat. Add 1 tablespoon of coconut oil to the skillet.
- Divide the ground beef into two equal portions and shape each into a patty.
- Season the patties with salt and pepper to taste.
- Place the patties in the skillet and cook for 3-4 minutes per side or until they are cooked to your liking.
- Remove the patties from the skillet and set them aside.
- Crack two eggs into the skillet and cook to your desired level of doneness.
- While the eggs are cooking, slice the avocado in half and remove the pit. Use a spoon to scoop the avocado out of the skin and slice it into thin pieces.
- Once the eggs are cooked, place them on a plate along with the beef patties and sliced avocado.
- Season the avocado with salt and pepper to taste.

BISON CHILI with AVOCADO and SOUR CREAM

What You Need

- 1 pound ground bison
- 1 onion, chopped
- 1 red bell pepper, chopped
- 3 cloves garlic, minced
- 1 tablespoon chili powder
- 1 teaspoon cumin
- 1/2 teaspoon smoked paprika
- 1/4 teaspoon cayenne pepper
- 1 can diced tomatoes (14.5 ounces)
- 1 can tomato sauce (8 ounces)
- 1/2 cup beef broth
- Salt and pepper, to taste
- Avocado, chopped green onions, and shredded cheese for topping (optional)

How To Cook

- In a large pot or Dutch oven over medium heat, brown the bison until no longer pink, breaking it up into small pieces with a spatula or spoon.
- Add the chopped onion, red bell pepper, and minced garlic to the pot and sauté until the vegetables are tender and the onion is translucent, about 5-7 minutes.
- Add the chili powder, cumin, smoked paprika, and cayenne pepper to the pot and stir to combine with the meat and vegetables.
- Pour in the can of diced tomatoes (with their juice), tomato sauce, and beef broth. Bring the mixture to a simmer, then reduce the heat to low and let the chili cook for at least 30 minutes, stirring occasionally.
- Season with salt and pepper to taste.
- Once the chili is cooked, serve it in bowls topped with avocado, chopped green onions, and shredded cheese if desired.

BRAISED SHORT RIBS with CAULIFLOWER MASHED

What You Need

Braised Short Ribs Ingredients:

- 1 pound beef short ribs
- 1 tablespoon grass-fed butter
- 1 tablespoon coconut oil or avocado oil
- 1/4 medium onion, diced
- 1 clove garlic, minced
- 1/2 cup beef broth
- 1 tablespoon tomato paste
- 1 tablespoon Worcestershire sauce
- 1/2 tablespoon chopped fresh rosemary
- Salt and pepper, to taste

Cauliflower Mashed Ingredients:

- 1/4 head cauliflower, cut into florets
- 1 tablespoon grass-fed butter
- 2 tablespoons heavy cream
- 2 tablespoons grated parmesan cheese
- Salt and pepper, to taste

How To Cook

- Preheat your oven to 325°F (163°C).
- Season the beef short ribs generously with salt and pepper.
- In a small oven-safe pot melt the butter and coconut oil or avocado oil over medium-high heat.
- Add the short ribs to the pot and sear on all sides until browned. Remove the short ribs, set aside.
- In the same pot, add the diced onion and minced garlic. Sauté until the onion is softened and golden.
- Add the beef broth, tomato paste, Worcestershire sauce, and chopped rosemary to the pot. and stir
- Return the short ribs to the pot, along with any accumulated juices. Bring the liquid to a boil.
- Cover the pot with a lid and transfer it to the preheated oven.
- Braise the short ribs in the oven for 2.5 to 3 hours, or until the meat is fork-tender and falling off the bone.
- Remove the pot from the oven and skim off any excess fat from the surface of the braising liquid.
- Place the pot back on the stovetop over medium heat. Simmer the braising liquid until it thickens and reduces to your desired consistency.

For the Cauliflower Mashed:

- While the short ribs are braising, prepare the cauliflower mashed.
- In a small pot, bring water to a boil. Add the cauliflower florets and cook until fork-tender, about 8-10 minutes.
- Drain the cauliflower and return it to the pot.
- Add the butter, heavy cream, grated parmesan cheese, to the pot with the cauliflower.
- Use an immersion blender or a potato masher to mash the cauliflower until smooth and creamy. Enjoy!

BROILED SALMON with ROASTED BRUSSELS SPROUTS and BACON

What You Need

- 2 salmon filets
- 1 tablespoon olive oil
- 1 teaspoon paprika
- 1 teaspoon garlic powder
- 1/2 teaspoon dried thyme
- Salt and pepper, to taste
- 1 pound Brussels sprouts, trimmed and halved
- 4 slices bacon, diced
- 1 tablespoon olive oil
- Salt and pepper, to taste

How To Cook

- Preheat the broiler to high.
- In a small bowl, mix together the olive oil, paprika, garlic powder, dried thyme, salt, and pepper.
- Brush the salmon filets with the spice mixture and place them on a baking sheet lined with parchment paper.
- Broil the salmon filets for 8-10 minutes, or until they are cooked through and lightly browned on top.
- While the salmon is broiling, preheat the oven to 400°F.
- Place the halved Brussels sprouts on a baking sheet lined with parchment paper.
- Drizzle the Brussels sprouts with olive oil and season with salt and pepper. Toss to coat evenly.
- Scatter the diced bacon over the Brussels sprouts.
- Roast the Brussels sprouts and bacon in the oven for 20-25 minutes, or until the Brussels sprouts are tender and the bacon is crispy.
- Serve the broiled salmon filets with the roasted Brussels sprouts and bacon on the side.
- Enjoy your delicious Broiled salmon with roasted Brussels sprouts and bacon!

BROILED SIRLOIN with CAULIFLOWER MASHED

What You Need

For the Sirloin Steak:
- 1 sirloin steak (8-10 oz)
- 2 tbsp butter
- 2 cloves garlic, minced
- Salt and pepper to taste

For the Cauliflower Mashed
- 1 small head of cauliflower
- 2 tbsp butter
- 1/4 cup heavy cream
- 1/4 cup grated parmesan cheese
- Salt and pepper to taste

How To Cook

- Prepare the Sirloin Steak:
- Remove the sirloin steak from the refrigerator and let it sit at room temperature for about 30 minutes before cooking.
- In a skillet over medium-high heat, melt the butter. Add the minced garlic and cook for 1-2 minutes until fragrant.
- Season the sirloin steak generously with salt and pepper on both sides.
- Place the steak in the skillet and sear for 3-4 minutes on each side for medium-rare, or longer for desired doneness.
- Once the steak is cooked to your liking, remove it from the skillet and let it rest for a few minutes before slicing.
- Prepare the Cauliflower Mash:
- In a large pot of boiling water, cook the cauliflower florets until fork-tender, about 8-10 minutes.
- Drain the cauliflower and return it to the pot.
- Add the butter, heavy cream, grated parmesan cheese, salt, and pepper to the pot with the cauliflower.
- Using an immersion blender or a potato masher, mash the cauliflower until it reaches your desired consistency. Taste and adjust seasoning as needed.
- Serve:
- Slice the rested sirloin steak against the grain into thin slices.
- Plate the sirloin steak alongside a generous serving of cauliflower mash.
- Enjoy your delicious and satisfying sirloin steak with creamy cauliflower mash.

BUFFALO CHICKEN LETTUCE WRAPS

What You Need

- 1 lb boneless, skinless chicken breasts, cooked and shredded
- 1/4 cup hot sauce
- 1/4 cup avocado mayonnaise
- 1/4 cup sour cream
- 1/4 tsp garlic powder
- Salt and pepper, to taste
- 8-10 large lettuce leaves
- Blue cheese crumbles, for topping
- Chopped celery, for topping

How To Cook

- In a mixing bowl, combine cooked and shredded chicken with hot sauce, avocado mayonnaise, sour cream, garlic powder, salt, and pepper. Mix well to combine.
- Take a large lettuce leaf and place 1-2 tablespoons of the chicken mixture in the center of the leaf.
- Top the chicken with blue cheese crumbles and chopped celery.
- Wrap the lettuce leaf around the chicken mixture to create a wrap.
- Repeat with remaining lettuce leaves and chicken mixture.
- Serve immediately and enjoy your delicious and low-carb Keto Buffalo Chicken Lettuce Wraps!

BUFFALO CHICKEN SALAD with BLUE CHEESE

What You Need

- 2 boneless, skinless chicken breasts
- 2 tbsp olive oil
- 1 tsp garlic powder
- 1 tsp onion powder
- 1 tsp paprika
- 1/4 tsp cayenne pepper
- Salt and pepper to taste
- 4 cups mixed greens
- 1/2 cup cherry tomatoes, halved
- 1/4 cup diced red onion
- 1/4 cup crumbled blue cheese
- 1/4 cup ranch dressing
- 1/4 cup Frank's RedHot sauce

How To Cook

- Preheat the oven to 400°F (200°C).
- In a small bowl, mix together the garlic powder, onion powder, paprika, cayenne pepper, salt, and pepper.
- Rub the chicken breasts with the olive oil, then coat them in the spice mixture.
- Place the chicken on a baking sheet and bake for 25-30 minutes, or until cooked through.
- Remove the chicken from the oven and let it cool for a few minutes. Then, cut it into bite-sized pieces.
- In a large bowl, combine the mixed greens, cherry tomatoes, and red onion.
- In a small bowl, whisk together the blue cheese dressing, hot sauce, and a pinch of salt.
- Add the chicken to the bowl with the salad ingredients and toss to combine.
- Drizzle the dressing over the top of the salad and serve.

BUFFALO WINGS with HOT SAUCE

What You Need

- 1 lb chicken wings, separated into drumettes and flats
- 1 tbsp baking powder
- 1 tsp salt
- 1/2 tsp black pepper
- 1/2 cup hot sauce (such as Frank's RedHot)
- 1/4 cup unsalted butter, melted
- 1/2 tsp garlic powder
- Celery sticks, for serving
- Blue cheese dressing, for serving

How To Cook

For the wings:

- Preheat the oven to 425°F.
- Line a baking sheet with foil and place a wire rack on top.
- In a small bowl, mix together the baking powder, salt, and black pepper.
- Pat the chicken wings dry with paper towels.
- Sprinkle the baking powder mixture over the wings and toss to coat evenly.
- Place the wings on the wire rack, making sure they are not touching.
- Bake the wings for 45-50 minutes, flipping them halfway through, until they are crispy and golden brown.

For the hot sauce:

- In a small saucepan, combine the hot sauce, melted butter, and garlic powder. Heat over low heat until the butter is melted and the ingredients are combined.
- Once the wings are done baking, toss them in the hot sauce until they are coated.
- Serve the hot wings with celery sticks and blue cheese dressing on the side.

BUTTER CHICKEN with CREAMY BROCCOLI

What You Need

For the Butter Chicken:

- 1 lb boneless, skinless chicken thighs, cut into bite-sized pieces
- 4 tbsp butter
- 1/2 cup diced onion
- 3 cloves garlic, minced
- 2 tbsp tomato paste
- 1 tbsp garam masala
- 1 tsp ground turmeric
- 1 tsp ground cumin
- 1/2 tsp paprika
- 1/4 tsp cayenne pepper (optional)
- 1/2 cup heavy cream
- Salt and pepper to taste
- Fresh cilantro for garnish (optional)

For the Creamy Broccoli with Bacon:

- 4 cups broccoli florets
- 4 slices bacon, cooked and crumbled
- 1/4 cup cream cheese
- 1/4 cup grated parmesan cheese
- Salt and pepper to taste

How To Cook

Prepare the Butter Chicken:

- In a large skillet over medium heat, melt the butter.
- Add the diced onion and minced garlic to the skillet and cook until softened, about 3-4 minutes.
- Add the chicken pieces to the skillet and cook until browned on all sides, about 5-6 minutes.
- Stir in the tomato paste, garam masala, turmeric, cumin, paprika, and cayenne pepper (if using) until well combined.
- Pour in the heavy cream and bring to a simmer. Let the sauce simmer for 5-7 minutes, stirring occasionally, until the chicken is cooked through and the sauce has thickened.
- Season with salt and pepper to taste. Garnish with fresh cilantro (optional).

Prepare the Creamy Broccoli with Bacon:

- In a separate pan, steam the broccoli florets until fork-tender, about 5-7 minutes.
- In a small saucepan over low heat, melt the cream cheese and grated parmesan cheese, stirring until smooth.
- Add the cooked and crumbled bacon to the saucepan with the melted cheese and stir until combined.

CHEESEBURGER CASSEROLE

What You Need

- 1 pound ground beef
- 1/2 onion, diced
- 1 can (14 oz) diced tomatoes
- 1 cup shredded cheddar cheese
- 4 eggs
- 1/2 cup heavy cream
- 1/4 cup unsweetened almond milk
- Salt and pepper to taste

How To Cook

- Preheat the oven to 350°F (175°C).
- In a large skillet, cook the ground beef and onion over medium-high heat until the beef is browned, breaking it up into smaller pieces as it cooks.
- Add the diced tomatoes, salt, and pepper to the skillet. Stir to combine and let it cook for a few minutes until the mixture thickens.
- Transfer the beef mixture to a greased 9x13 inch baking dish.
- Sprinkle the shredded cheddar cheese over the beef mixture.
- In a separate bowl, whisk together the eggs, heavy cream, and almond milk. Pour the mixture over the cheese and beef mixture in the baking dish.
- Bake in the preheated oven for 30-35 minutes until the casserole is golden brown and the eggs are set.
- Let cool for a few minutes before serving. Enjoy!

CHICKEN BONE BROTH with GINGER and TURMERIC

What You Need

- 2-3 pounds of chicken bones (with or without meat)
- 1 onion, peeled and roughly chopped
- 2 carrots, roughly chopped
- 2 celery stalks, roughly chopped
- 4 cloves garlic, peeled and smashed
- 1 knob ginger, peeled and roughly chopped
- 1 knob turmeric, peeled and roughly chopped (or 1 tsp turmeric powder)
- 2 bay leaves
- 1 tablespoon apple cider vinegar
- Salt and pepper, to taste
- Water, enough to cover the bones and vegetables

How To Cook

- Preheat your oven to 400°F (200°C).
- Spread the chicken bones (with or without meat) on a baking sheet and roast for 30 minutes, flipping halfway through.
- Meanwhile, in a large stockpot or Dutch oven, add the chopped onion, carrots, celery, garlic, ginger, turmeric, and bay leaves.
- Add the roasted chicken bones and any juices from the baking sheet to the pot.
- Pour enough water into the pot to cover the bones and vegetables (about 8-10 cups).
- Add the apple cider vinegar and season with salt and pepper to taste.
- Bring the mixture to a boil over high heat, then reduce the heat to low and let it simmer for 8-12 hours.
- After simmering, strain the broth through a fine-mesh strainer or cheesecloth to remove the solids.
- Let the broth cool and store it in an airtight container in the refrigerator for up to 5 days, or in the freezer for up to 6 months.

CHICKEN BREAST with ZUCCHINI

What You Need

For the chicken:

- 2 boneless, skinless chicken breasts
- 2 tbsp. olive oil
- 1 tbsp. butter
- 1 tbsp. minced garlic
- Salt and pepper, to taste
- 1 tbsp. fresh parsley, chopped

For the roasted zucchini:

- 2 medium zucchinis, sliced into rounds
- 2 tbsp. olive oil
- 1 tsp. garlic powder
- Salt and pepper, to taste
- 1/4 cup grated Parmesan cheese (optional)

How To Cook

- Preheat your oven to 400°F.
- Place the chicken breasts in a baking dish, and season both sides with salt and pepper.
- In a small bowl, mix together the olive oil, butter, and minced garlic. Spoon the mixture over the chicken breasts, making sure they are coated evenly.
- Bake the chicken in the preheated oven for 25-30 minutes, or until the internal temperature reaches 165°F.
- While the chicken is cooking, prepare the roasted zucchini. Place the sliced zucchini in a large mixing bowl.
- Drizzle the zucchini with olive oil and sprinkle with garlic powder, salt, and pepper. Toss to coat the zucchini evenly.
- Spread the zucchini out on a baking sheet lined with parchment paper.
- Roast the zucchini in the preheated oven for 20-25 minutes, or until it is lightly browned.
- Once the chicken is cooked, remove it from the oven and let it rest for 5-10 minutes before slicing.
- Serve the chicken with the roasted zucchini on the side, and sprinkle with fresh chopped parsley for garnish.

CHICKEN CAESAR SALAD

What You Need

- 2 chicken breasts
- Salt and pepper, to taste
- 4 cups romaine lettuce, chopped
- 1/4 cup grated Parmesan cheese
- 2 tablespoons olive oil
- 1 tablespoon lemon juice
- 1 tablespoon Dijon mustard
- 1 clove garlic, minced
- 1/4 teaspoon Worcestershire sauce
- 1/4 teaspoon anchovy paste (optional)

How To Cook

- Preheat the oven to 375°F (190°C).
- Season the chicken breasts with salt and pepper to taste. Place them on a baking sheet and bake in the preheated oven for 20-25 minutes, or until cooked through.
- Let the chicken cool for a few minutes, then chop it into bite-sized pieces.
- In a large bowl, combine the chopped romaine lettuce and grated Parmesan cheese.
- In a small bowl, whisk together the olive oil, lemon juice, Dijon mustard, minced garlic, Worcestershire sauce, and anchovy paste (if using).
- Pour the dressing over the romaine lettuce and toss to coat.
- Top the salad with the chopped chicken.
- Serve immediately.
- This Chicken Caesar Salad is a delicious and satisfying lunch or dinner option that's packed with protein and healthy fats. It's also easy to make and can be customized with additional toppings such as bacon, avocado, or cherry tomatoes. Enjoy!

COBB SALAD with HAMBURGER PATTY

What You Need

For the salad:

- 4 cups mixed salad greens
- 1/2 cup cooked and crumbled bacon
- 1/2 cup crumbled blue cheese or feta cheese
- 1/2 cup cherry tomatoes, halved
- 1/2 cup diced cooked chicken breast
- 1/2 avocado, diced
- 4 hard-boiled eggs, peeled and halved
- 1 hamburger patty, cooked to your desired level of doneness

For the dressing:

- 1/4 cup olive oil
- 2 tablespoons red wine vinegar
- 1 tablespoon Dijon mustard
- 1 clove garlic, minced
- Salt and black pepper to taste

How To Cook

- Prepare all the salad ingredients by washing and drying the salad greens, cooking the bacon, crumbling the cheese, halving the cherry tomatoes, dicing the cooked chicken breast, and peeling and halving the hard-boiled eggs.
- Season the hamburger patty with salt and black pepper, and cook it to your desired level of doneness using your preferred method (grilling, stovetop, etc.). Set aside.
- In a small bowl, whisk together the olive oil, red wine vinegar, Dijon mustard, minced garlic, salt, and black pepper to make the dressing.
- In a large salad bowl, arrange the mixed salad greens. Arrange the cooked bacon, crumbled cheese, cherry tomatoes, diced chicken breast, diced avocado, and hard-boiled eggs on top of the salad greens.
- Place the cooked hamburger patty on top of the salad.
- Drizzle the dressing over the salad and hamburger patty.
-

COCONUT CURRY CHICKEN with CAULIFLOWER RICE

What You Need

- 2 boneless, skinless chicken breasts, diced
- 1 tablespoon coconut oil or ghee
- 1/2 medium onion, chopped
- 2 cloves garlic, minced
- 1 tablespoon curry powder
- 1/2 teaspoon turmeric
- 1/2 teaspoon cumin
- 1/2 teaspoon paprika
- 1/4 teaspoon cayenne pepper
- 1/4 teaspoon salt
- 1/4 teaspoon black pepper
- 1 can (13.5 oz) coconut milk (full-fat)
- 1/2 cup chicken broth
- 1/2 cup diced tomatoes (canned or fresh)
- 1/2 cup chopped bell peppers
- 1/2 cup chopped zucchini
- 1/2 cup chopped mushrooms

For Cauliflower Rice

- 1 small head of cauliflower, riced
- 2 tablespoons coconut oil
- Salt and pepper to taste

How To Cook

- In a large skillet over medium heat, melt the coconut oil or ghee. Add the chopped onion and minced garlic and sauté until softened and fragrant, about 2-3 minutes.
- Add the diced chicken breasts to the skillet and cook until browned on all sides, about 5-6 minutes.
- Add the curry powder, turmeric, cumin, paprika, cayenne pepper (if using), salt, and black pepper to the skillet. Stir to coat the chicken and vegetables in the spices.
- Pour in the coconut milk, chicken broth, diced tomatoes, chopped bell peppers, zucchini, and mushrooms. Bring to a simmer and let it cook for about 10-12 minutes, or until the chicken is cooked through and the vegetables are tender.
- Stir in the fish sauce (if using) for an extra umami flavor. Taste and adjust seasoning as needed.
- Meanwhile, prepare the cauliflower rice. Using a food processor or box grater, grate the cauliflower into rice-like pieces.
- In a separate skillet over medium heat, melt the coconut oil or ghee. Add the riced cauliflower and sauté for 5-6 minutes, or until it reaches your desired level of tenderness. Season with salt and pepper to taste.

COCONUT CURRY SHRIMP with CAULIFLOWER RICE

What You Need

For the Coconut Curry Shrimp:

- 1 lb large shrimp, peeled and deveined
- 2 tbsp coconut oil
- 1/2 cup diced onion
- 3 cloves garlic, minced
- 2 tbsp red curry paste
- 1 can (13.5 oz) coconut milk (full-fat)
- 1 tbsp fish sauce
- 1 tbsp lime juice
- 1 tbsp erythritol or preferred keto-friendly sweetener
- Salt and pepper to taste
- Fresh cilantro for garnish (optional)

For the Cauliflower Rice:

1 small head of cauliflower, riced

2 tbsp coconut oil

Salt and pepper to taste

How To Cook

- Prepare the Coconut Curry Shrimp:
- In a large skillet over medium heat, melt the coconut oil.
- Add the diced onion and minced garlic to the skillet and cook until softened, about 3-4 minutes.
- Add the red curry paste to the skillet and cook for an additional 1-2 minutes, stirring constantly.
- Add the shrimp to the skillet and cook until pink and opaque, about 3-4 minutes per side.
- Stir in the coconut milk, fish sauce, lime juice, and erythritol (or preferred keto-friendly sweetener) until well combined.
- Let the curry simmer for 5-7 minutes, stirring occasionally, to allow the flavors to meld together.
- Season with salt and pepper to taste. Garnish with fresh cilantro (optional).
- Prepare the Cauliflower Rice:
- In a separate pan, heat the coconut oil over medium heat.
- Add the riced cauliflower to the pan and cook for 5-7 minutes, stirring occasionally, until the cauliflower is tender but not mushy.
- Season with salt and pepper to taste. Enjoy!

EGGPLANT PARMESAN

What You Need

- 1 large eggplant, sliced into rounds
- 2 cups almond flour
- 2 tsp garlic powder
- 2 tsp onion powder
- 1 tsp salt
- 1/2 tsp black pepper
- 2 eggs, whisked
- 1 cup marinara sauce
- 2 cups shredded mozzarella cheese
- 1/2 cup grated parmesan cheese
- Fresh basil leaves for garnish

How To Cook

- Preheat the oven to 375°F (190°C).
- In a shallow bowl, combine almond flour, garlic powder, onion powder, salt, and black pepper.
- Dip eggplant rounds into the whisked eggs, then coat with the almond flour mixture. Repeat until all eggplant slices are coated.
- Place the coated eggplant slices on a baking sheet lined with parchment paper.
- Bake in the preheated oven for 25-30 minutes, until the eggplant is tender and the coating is golden brown.
- Remove the eggplant from the oven and spread a thin layer of marinara sauce over each slice.
- Sprinkle shredded mozzarella cheese and grated parmesan cheese over the marinara sauce.
- Return the eggplant to the oven and bake for an additional 10-15 minutes, until the cheese is melted and bubbly.
- Remove from the oven and let cool for a few minutes before serving.
- Garnish with fresh basil leaves and serve hot.
- Enjoy your delicious and healthy Keto Eggplant Parmesan!

FETA STUFFED CHICKEN BREAST with CAULIFLOWER MASHED

What You Need

- 4 boneless, skinless chicken breasts
- 2 cups spinach, chopped
- 1/2 cup crumbled feta cheese
- 1/4 cup cream cheese, softened
- 2 cloves garlic, minced
- 1/4 teaspoon dried oregano
- 1/4 teaspoon dried basil
- 1/4 teaspoon salt
- 1/4 teaspoon black pepper
- 2 tablespoons olive oil or melted butter for brushing
- 4 cups cauliflower florets
- 2 tablespoons butter
- Salt and pepper to taste

How To Cook

- Preheat your oven to 375°F (190°C).
- In a mixing bowl, combine the chopped spinach, crumbled feta cheese, softened cream cheese, minced garlic, dried oregano, dried basil, salt, and black pepper. Mix well to form a stuffing mixture.
- Butterfly each chicken breast by slicing horizontally through the center, leaving one edge intact to create a pocket for the stuffing.
- Stuff each chicken breast with a generous spoonful of the spinach and feta mixture, then close the pocket and secure with toothpicks if needed.
- Place the stuffed chicken breasts on a baking sheet or in a baking dish. Brush the tops with olive oil or melted butter for added richness.
- Bake the stuffed chicken breasts in the preheated oven for 25-30 minutes, or until the internal temperature reaches 165°F (74°C) and the chicken is cooked through.
- While the chicken is baking, prepare the cauliflower mashed. Steam or boil the cauliflower florets until fork-tender, then drain well.
- In a blender or food processor, combine the cooked cauliflower, butter, salt, and pepper. Blend until smooth and creamy, adjusting seasoning to taste.
- Once the chicken breasts are cooked, remove them from the oven and let them rest for a few minutes before serving. Enjoy!

GARLIC BUTTER PORK TENDERLOIN with ASPARAGUS

What You Need

For the Garlic Pork Tenderloin:

- 1 lb pork tenderloin
- 4 cloves garlic, minced
- 2 tbsp butter
- 1 tbsp olive oil
- Salt and pepper to taste
- Fresh rosemary or thyme for garnish (optional)

For the Asparagus:

- 1 lb asparagus, trimmed
- 2 tbsp butter
- 2 cloves garlic, minced
- Salt and pepper to taste
- Lemon wedges for serving (optional)

How To Cook

- Prepare the Garlic Pork Tenderloin:
- Preheat your oven to 400°F (200°C).
- Season the pork tenderloin with salt and pepper on all sides.
- In an oven-safe skillet over medium-high heat, melt the butter and olive oil.
- Add the minced garlic to the skillet and cook until fragrant, about 1 minute.
- Add the seasoned pork tenderloin to the skillet and sear on all sides until browned, about 2-3 minutes per side.
- Transfer the skillet to the preheated oven and bake for 15-20 minutes, or until the internal temperature of the pork reaches 145°F (63°C).
- Remove the skillet from the oven and let the pork tenderloin rest for a few minutes before slicing. Garnish with fresh rosemary or thyme (optional).
- Prepare the Asparagus:
- While the pork tenderloin is resting, prepare the asparagus.
- In a separate pan over medium heat, melt the butter.
- Add the minced garlic to the pan and cook until fragrant, about 1 minute.
- Add the trimmed asparagus to the pan and cook for 5-7 minutes, stirring occasionally, until the asparagus is tender but still crisp.
- Season with salt and pepper to taste. Enjoy!

GARLIC BUTTER STEAK BITES with EGGS and BACON

What You Need

- 1 pound sirloin steak, cut into bite-sized pieces
- 4 tablespoons butter
- 4 cloves garlic, minced
- Salt and black pepper, to taste
- 4 slices bacon, diced
- 4 eggs

How To Cook

- Preheat a large skillet over medium-high heat.
- Season the steak bites generously with salt and black pepper.
- Add 2 tablespoons of butter to the skillet and let it melt.
- Add the steak bites to the skillet and cook for about 2-3 minutes per side or until browned and cooked to your liking.
- Remove the steak bites from the skillet and set aside.
- In the same skillet, add the remaining 2 tablespoons of butter and let it melt.
- Add the minced garlic and cook for about 30 seconds, stirring constantly.
- Add the diced bacon to the skillet and cook until crispy, stirring occasionally.
- Remove the bacon from the skillet and set aside.
- Crack the eggs into the skillet and cook to your liking, seasoning with salt and black pepper.
- Serve the steak bites with the garlic butter sauce drizzled on top, alongside the eggs and bacon.
- Enjoy your high fat garlic butter steak bites with eggs and bacon!

GRILLED CHICKEN with ROASTED ASPARAGUS and MUSHROOMS

What You Need

- 2 chicken thighs
- 1 tablespoon olive oil
- Salt and pepper, to taste
- 1/2 teaspoon garlic powder
- 1/2 teaspoon onion powder
- 1/2 teaspoon paprika
- 1/2 teaspoon dried thyme
- 1/2 teaspoon dried rosemary
- 1/2 pound asparagus
- 1 cup mushrooms, sliced
- 2 tablespoons butter
- Lemon wedges, for serving

How To Cook

- Preheat a grill to medium-high heat.
- In a small bowl, mix together the garlic powder, onion powder, paprika, thyme, and rosemary.
- Rub the chicken thighs with olive oil, then season them with the spice mixture, salt, and pepper.
- Grill the chicken thighs for 6-8 minutes per side, or until the internal temperature reaches 165°F.
- While the chicken is grilling, preheat the oven to 400°F.
- Place the asparagus and mushrooms on a baking sheet lined with parchment paper.
- Drizzle the vegetables with olive oil and season with salt and pepper.
- Roast the vegetables in the oven for 15-20 minutes, or until they are tender and lightly browned.
- In a small saucepan, melt the butter over medium heat.
- Serve the grilled chicken with the roasted asparagus and mushrooms, drizzled with melted butter and garnished with lemon wedges.

GRILLED SALMON with ASPARAGUS and LEMON

What You Need

- 6 oz salmon filet
- 1/2 tbsp olive oil
- Salt and black pepper, to taste
- 6 spears of asparagus
- 1/2 lemon

How To Cook

- Preheat a grill pan over medium-high heat.
- Brush the salmon filet with olive oil on both sides and season generously with salt and black pepper.
- Place the salmon filet on the grill pan, skin side down, and cook for about 5-6 minutes.
- While the salmon is cooking, prepare the asparagus. Trim the ends and toss with olive oil, salt, and black pepper.
- After 5-6 minutes, flip the salmon filet over and add the asparagus to the grill pan. Cook for another 4-5 minutes or until the salmon is cooked through and the asparagus is tender.
- Remove the salmon and asparagus from the grill pan and transfer to a plate.
- Squeeze half a lemon over the salmon and asparagus.
- Drizzle some additional olive oil on top for extra fat.
- Enjoy your grilled salmon with asparagus and lemon!

GRILLED SARDINES with LEMON and OLIVE OIL

What You Need

- 8 fresh sardines, cleaned and scaled
- 2 lemons, sliced
- 1/4 cup olive oil
- 2 cloves garlic, minced
- Salt and pepper, to taste

How To Cook

- Preheat your grill to medium-high heat.
- Rinse the sardines under cold running water and pat them dry with paper towels.
- In a small bowl, whisk together the olive oil, minced garlic, salt, and pepper.
- Brush the sardines with the olive oil mixture, making sure to coat them evenly.
- Place the sardines on the grill, flesh side down. Grill for 3-4 minutes, or until the flesh is lightly charred and the skin is crispy.
- Carefully flip the sardines over using a spatula or tongs. Grill for an additional 2-3 minutes, or until the second side is lightly charred and the flesh is cooked through.
- Transfer the grilled sardines to a serving platter and squeeze fresh lemon juice over the top.
- Garnish with lemon slices and serve hot.
- Enjoy your delicious and healthy grilled sardines with lemon and olive oil!

GRILLED TROUT with ASPARAGUS

What You Need

For the trout:

- 2 fresh trout filets
- 1 tbsp. olive oil
- 1 tbsp. fresh parsley, chopped
- 1 tbsp. fresh thyme, chopped
- Salt and pepper, to taste
- Lemon wedges, for serving

For the asparagus:

- 1 bunch asparagus, ends trimmed
- 1 tbsp. olive oil
- Salt and pepper, to taste

How To Cook

- Preheat the grill to medium-high heat.
- In a small bowl, mix together the olive oil, parsley, thyme, salt, and pepper.
- Brush the trout filets with the herb mixture, making sure to coat both sides.
- Place the trout filets on the grill, skin-side down. Cook for 5-7 minutes, or until the skin is crispy and the fish is cooked through.
- While the trout is cooking, prepare the asparagus. Place the asparagus on a baking sheet and drizzle with olive oil. Season with salt and pepper.
- Place the baking sheet in the oven and roast the asparagus for 10-15 minutes, or until they are tender and lightly browned.
- Once the trout and asparagus are done, serve them together on a plate. Squeeze a lemon wedge over the trout before serving.
- Enjoy your delicious and healthy grilled trout with herb and roasted asparagus!

KETO BAKED EGGS FLORENTINE

What You Need

- 4 large eggs
- 2 cups fresh spinach leaves
- 1/2 cup heavy cream
- 1/2 cup shredded mozzarella cheese
- 1/4 cup grated parmesan cheese
- 2 tbsp butter
- 1 tbsp nutritional yeast
- 1/2 tsp garlic powder
- 1/2 tsp onion powder
- Salt and pepper to taste
- Optional: chopped fresh herbs (such as parsley or chives) for garnish

How To Cook

- Preheat your oven to 375°F (190°C) and grease four ramekins or oven-safe dishes.
- In a skillet over medium heat, melt the butter. Add the fresh spinach leaves and cook until wilted, stirring occasionally.
- In a small bowl, whisk together the heavy cream, garlic powder, onion powder, nutritional yeast, salt, and pepper.
- Place a layer of wilted spinach in the bottom of each greased ramekin or oven-safe dish.
- Pour about 1-2 tablespoons of the cream mixture over the spinach in each ramekin.
- Crack one egg into each ramekin, making sure not to break the yolk.
- Top each ramekin with shredded mozzarella cheese and grated parmesan cheese.
- Bake in the preheated oven for 12-15 minutes or until the whites are set but the yolks are still slightly runny.
- Remove from the oven and let the baked eggs florentine cool for a few minutes before serving.
- Enjoy!

KETO BREAD

What You Need

- 1 1/2 cups almond flour
- 6 large eggs, separated
- 1/4 cup unsalted butter, melted
- 1/4 tsp cream of tartar
- 1/2 tsp baking powder
- 1/4 tsp salt

How To Cook

- Preheat your oven to 325°F (160°C) and line a 9x5-inch loaf pan with parchment paper.
- In a large mixing bowl, whisk together the almond flour, egg yolks, melted butter, baking powder, and salt until well combined.
- In a separate bowl, beat the egg whites and cream of tartar with an electric mixer on high speed until stiff peaks form.
- Gently fold the beaten egg whites into the almond flour mixture until just combined, being careful not to deflate the egg whites.
- Pour the batter into the prepared loaf pan and smooth the top with a spatula.
- Bake in the preheated oven for 35-40 minutes or until a toothpick inserted into the center comes out clean.
- Remove the bread from the oven and let it cool in the pan for 10 minutes, then transfer to a wire rack to cool completely.
- Once cooled, slice the bread into desired thickness and serve as a sandwich bread, toast, or with your favorite keto-friendly spreads.
- Note: You can customize the flavor of your keto bread by adding herbs, spices, cheese, or other low-carb ingredients to the batter. Store the leftover bread in an airtight container in the refrigerator for up to 5 days or in the freezer for longer storage. Toasting the slices before serving can enhance the flavor and texture of the bread.

KETO BREAKFAST CASSEROLE

What You Need

- 8 large eggs
- 1/2 cup heavy cream
- 1/2 cup diced bell peppers (any color)
- 1/2 cup diced onions
- 1 cup shredded cheese (cheddar, mozzarella, or your preferred cheese)
- 1 tablespoon unfortified nutritional yeast
- 1/2 teaspoon salt
- 1/4 teaspoon black pepper
- 2 tablespoons olive oil (for drizzling)
- 1 tablespoon grass fed butter.

How To Cook

- Preheat your oven to 350°F (175°C) and grease a 9x9-inch baking dish with grass fed butter.
- In a large bowl, whisk together the eggs, heavy cream, nutritional yeast, salt, and black pepper.
- Stir in the diced bell peppers, onions, and shredded cheese into the egg mixture.
- Pour the mixture into the greased baking dish and spread it out evenly.
- Drizzle olive oil over the top of the casserole.
- Bake in the preheated oven for 25-30 minutes or until the eggs are set and the top is golden brown.
- Remove from the oven and let the casserole cool slightly before serving.
- Add some slices of butter on top.
- Cut into slices or squares and serve hot as a delicious and satisfying breakfast casserole. Enjoy!

KETO TUNA SALAD CUPS

What You Need

For the tuna salad:

- 1 can tuna, drained
- 1/4 cup mayonnaise
- 1/4 cup diced celery
- 2 tbsp diced red onion
- 2 tbsp chopped fresh parsley
- 1 tsp dijon mustard
- Salt and pepper to taste

For the salad cups:

- Lettuce leaves, such as butter lettuce, romaine, or iceberg
- Optional toppings: sliced avocado, cherry tomatoes, cucumber slices, olives, etc.

How To Cook

- In a medium bowl, mix together the drained tuna, avocado mayonnaise, diced celery, diced red onion, chopped parsley, dijon mustard, salt, and pepper until well combined.
- Taste and adjust seasoning as desired.
- Wash and dry the lettuce leaves, and arrange them on a serving platter or individual plates to form cups.
- Spoon the tuna salad into the lettuce cups.
- Add any optional toppings, such as sliced avocado, cherry tomatoes, cucumber slices, or olives.
- Serve the keto tuna salad cups as a refreshing and low-carb appetizer, lunch, or light dinner.

LAMB CHOPS with ROASTED ASPARAGUS

What You Need

For the lamb chops:

- 4-6 lamb chops
- 1 tablespoon olive oil
- 1 tablespoon fresh rosemary, chopped
- 1 tablespoon fresh thyme, chopped
- 2 cloves garlic, minced
- Salt and pepper, to taste

For the roasted asparagus:

- 1 lb fresh asparagus, trimmed
- 2 tablespoons olive oil
- 2 cloves garlic, minced
- Salt and pepper, to taste

How To Cook

- Preheat your oven to 400°F.
- In a small bowl, mix together the olive oil, chopped rosemary, chopped thyme, minced garlic, salt, and pepper.
- Rub the herb mixture all over the lamb chops, making sure to coat them evenly.
- Heat a large oven-safe skillet over medium-high heat. Once hot, add the lamb chops and sear them on all sides until browned, about 2-3 minutes per side.
- Transfer the skillet to the preheated oven and bake the lamb chops for 10-15 minutes, or until they are cooked to your liking. For medium-rare, the internal temperature should be around 145°F.
- While the lamb chops are cooking, prepare the roasted asparagus. Place the trimmed asparagus on a baking sheet lined with parchment paper.
- Drizzle the asparagus with olive oil and sprinkle with minced garlic, salt, and pepper. Toss to coat the asparagus evenly.
- Roast the asparagus in the preheated oven for 10-15 minutes, or until they are tender and lightly charred.
- Once the lamb chops are cooked, remove the skillet from the oven.

LAMB MEATBALLS with CAULIFLOWER RICE and SAUCE

What You Need

- 1 pound ground lamb
- 1/2 cup almond flour
- 1/4 cup fresh parsley, chopped
- 2 cloves garlic, minced
- 1 egg
- Salt and pepper, to taste
- 1 head cauliflower, grated or processed into rice-sized pieces
- 1/4 cup olive oil
- 1/2 cup onion, chopped
- 2 cloves garlic, minced
- 1 can (14 ounces) diced tomatoes, undrained
- 1 teaspoon dried oregano
- 1 teaspoon dried basil
- Salt and pepper, to taste

How To Cook

- Preheat the oven to 400°F.
- In a large bowl, combine the ground lamb, almond flour, chopped parsley, minced garlic, egg, salt, and pepper. Mix well.
- Shape the lamb mixture into 12-16 meatballs, about 2 inches in diameter.
- Place the meatballs on a baking sheet lined with parchment paper and bake in the oven for 15-20 minutes, or until they are browned and cooked through.
- While the meatballs are cooking, heat the olive oil in a large skillet over medium heat.
- Add the chopped onion and minced garlic to the skillet and sauté for 2-3 minutes, until the onion is translucent.
- Add the diced tomatoes, dried oregano, dried basil, salt, and pepper to the skillet. Stir well to combine.
- Reduce the heat to low and simmer the tomato sauce for 10-15 minutes, until it has thickened and the flavors have melded together.
- While the tomato sauce is simmering, prepare the cauliflower rice by heating a separate skillet over medium heat.
- Add the grated or processed cauliflower rice to the skillet and sauté for 3-4 minutes, until it is tender and lightly browned. Enjoy!

LEMON GARLIC SHRIMP with ZUCCHINI NOODLES

What You Need

- 1 pound large shrimp, peeled and deveined
- 3 cloves garlic, minced
- 1 tablespoon olive oil
- Salt and pepper
- Juice of 1 lemon
- Zest of 1 lemon
- 2 medium zucchini, spiralized into noodles
- 2 tablespoons chopped fresh parsley

How To Cook

- Heat a large skillet over medium-high heat. Add the olive oil and let it heat up for 1-2 minutes.
- Add the minced garlic to the skillet and sauté for 1-2 minutes until fragrant.
- Add the shrimp to the skillet and season with a pinch of salt and pepper. Cook for 2-3 minutes until the shrimp are pink and cooked through.
- Add the lemon juice and zest to the skillet and toss to coat the shrimp evenly.
- Add the zucchini noodles to the skillet and toss to combine with the shrimp and garlic. Cook for 1-2 minutes until the zucchini noodles are tender.
- Remove the skillet from the heat and garnish with chopped parsley.
- Serve immediately, and enjoy your delicious Lemon Garlic Shrimp with Zucchini Noodles!
- Optional: If desired, you can add a side of roasted Brussels sprouts or steamed broccoli to complete the meal.

LETTUCE WRAPPED CHEESEBURGERS

What You Need

- 1 pound ground beef
- 4-6 leaves of iceberg lettuce
- 4 slices of bacon
- 1 ripe avocado, sliced
- 4 slices of cheddar cheese
- Salt and pepper, to taste

How To Cook

- Preheat your grill or a large skillet over medium-high heat.
- Divide the ground beef into 4 equal portions and shape them into patties. Season each patty with salt and pepper on both sides.
- Cook the bacon until crispy and set it aside.
- Grill or cook the beef patties for about 3-5 minutes per side, or until they are cooked to your desired level of doneness.
- Place a slice of cheddar cheese on top of each patty and allow it to melt.
- Wash the lettuce leaves and pat them dry. Use them as a replacement for traditional hamburger buns.
- Place the lettuce leaves on plates and add the beef patties on top of each leaf.
- Add the sliced avocado and bacon on top of the beef patties.
- Serve immediately and enjoy!
- This recipe is easy to customize to your own taste. Feel free to add your favorite toppings or condiments, such as onion or pickles

MEAT LOVERS FRITTATA

What You Need

- 8 large eggs
- 1/4 cup heavy cream
- 1/4 cup grated Parmesan cheese
- 1/2 tsp salt
- 1/4 tsp black pepper
- 1 tbsp olive oil
- 1/2 cup chopped onion
- 1/2 cup chopped green bell pepper
- 4 oz cooked bacon, chopped
- 4 oz cooked sausage, crumbled
- 4 oz cooked ham, chopped
- 1/2 cup shredded cheddar cheese
- Fresh parsley, chopped (optional)

How To Cook

- Preheat the oven to 375°F (190°C).
- In a large mixing bowl, whisk together eggs, heavy cream, Parmesan cheese, salt, and black pepper.
- In a 10-inch oven-safe skillet, heat olive oil over medium heat. Add onion and green bell pepper and cook until softened, about 5 minutes.
- Add the bacon, sausage, and ham to the skillet and stir to combine.
- Pour the egg mixture over the meat and vegetables in the skillet. Use a spatula to distribute everything evenly.
- Sprinkle shredded cheddar cheese over the top of the frittata.
- Transfer the skillet to the preheated oven and bake for 20-25 minutes or until the frittata is set in the center and the cheese is melted and bubbly.
- Remove the skillet from the oven and let the frittata cool for a few minutes.
- Garnish with fresh chopped parsley (optional).
- Slice the frittata into wedges and serve hot.
- Enjoy your delicious high meat lovers frittata!

MEAT LOVERS OMELET with AVOCADO

What You Need

- 4 large eggs
- 1/4 cup heavy cream
- 1/4 teaspoon salt
- 1/4 teaspoon black pepper
- 1 tablespoon nutritional yeast
- 2 tablespoons grass-fed butter
- 2 slices bacon, cooked and crumbled
- 2 sausage links, cooked and sliced
- 1/4 cup diced ham
- 1/4 cup shredded cheddar cheese
- 1/4 avocado, sliced

How To Cook

- In a bowl, whisk together the eggs, heavy cream, salt, and black pepper and nutritional yeast until well combined.
- Heat a skillet over medium heat and melt the grass-fed butter.
- Pour the egg mixture into the skillet and swirl it around to coat the whole pan.
- Cook the eggs for 2-3 minutes, lifting the edges with a spatula and tilting the skillet to allow the uncooked eggs to flow underneath, until the eggs are set but still slightly soft on top.
- Sprinkle the cooked bacon, sausage, ham, and shredded cheddar cheese over one half of the omelet.
- Carefully fold the other half of the omelet over the filling to create a half-moon shape.
- Cook for another 1-2 minutes, or until the cheese is melted and the filling is heated through.
- Slide the omelet onto a plate and top with sliced avocado.
- Enjoy your delicious high-fat keto meat lovers omelet with avocado!

MEATLOAF MASHED GREEN BEANS

What You Need

Meatloaf Ingredients:

- 1 pound ground beef
- 1/2 cup almond flour
- 1/2 cup grated Parmesan cheese
- 1/2 cup diced onions
- 1/2 cup diced bell peppers (any color)
- 2 large eggs
- 2 tablespoons tomato paste
- 2 tablespoons Worcestershire sauce
- 1 teaspoon garlic powder
- 1 teaspoon onion powder
- 1/2 teaspoon dried oregano
- 1/2 teaspoon dried basil
- 1/2 teaspoon salt
- 1/4 teaspoon black pepper
- 2 tablespoons grass-fed butter (melted)
- Olive oil (for brushing)

Cauliflower Mash Ingredients:

- 1 small head cauliflower, cut
- 4 tablespoons grass-fed butter
- Salt and pepper to taste

Green Beans Ingredients:

- 1 pound green beans, trimmed
- 2 tablespoons olive oil
- Salt and pepper to taste

How To Cook

- Preheat your oven to 375°F (190°C) and grease a loaf pan.
- In a large bowl, combine the ground beef, almond flour, Parmesan cheese, diced onions, diced bell peppers, eggs, tomato paste, Worcestershire sauce, garlic powder, onion powder, dried oregano, dried basil, salt, pepper, and melted grass-fed butter. Mix well.
- Press the meatloaf mixture into the greased loaf pan, shaping it into a loaf shape.
- Brush the top of the meatloaf with olive oil to help with browning.
- Bake in the preheated oven for 45-50 minutes. Meanwhile, prepare the cauliflower mash by boiling the cauliflower florets in a pot of salted water until fork-tender. Drain the cauliflower and transfer it to a food processor or blender.
- Add the grass-fed butter, salt, and pepper to the cauliflower and blend until smooth and creamy.
- In a separate pan, heat olive oil over medium heat. Add the trimmed green beans and sauté for 5-7 minutes, until they are tender but still crisp. Season with salt and pepper to taste.
- Once the meatloaf is cooked, remove it from the oven and let it rest for a few minutes before slicing. Enjoy!

NEW YORK STEAK and EGGS with BACON

What You Need

- 1 New York steak (12-16 oz)
- 4 slices of bacon
- 4 large eggs
- 1/2 cup shredded cheese (e.g. cheddar, gouda, or your favorite cheese)
- 1 tablespoon nutritional yeast
- Salt and pepper to taste
- Butter or cooking oil for cooking

How To Cook

- Season the New York steak generously with salt and pepper on both sides. Let it sit at room temperature for about 30 minutes to come to room temperature.
- In a large skillet over medium-high heat, cook the bacon until crispy. Remove the cooked bacon slices from the skillet and set aside.
- In the same skillet with the bacon grease, add some butter or cooking oil if needed. Add the New York steak to the skillet and cook to your desired level of doneness. For medium-rare, cook for about 4-5 minutes per side, depending on the thickness of the steak. Adjust cooking time for your preferred level of doneness.
- Once the steak is cooked to your liking, remove it from the skillet and let it rest for a few minutes before slicing.
- In the same skillet with the remaining bacon grease and steak drippings, crack the eggs into the skillet and cook to your desired level of doneness. You can fry them sunny-side up, over easy, or however you prefer.
- Sprinkle the shredded cheese and nutritional yeast over the eggs in the skillet and cover with a lid to melt the cheese and warm the nutritional yeast.
- Arrange the cooked New York steak, bacon slices, and cheesy eggs on a serving plate.
- Serve hot and enjoy your high-fat New York steak and eggs with bacon, cheese, and nutritional yeast!

NEW YORK STEAK with BACON WRAPPED GREEN BEANS

What You Need

For the New York Steak:

- 1 New York steak, about 8-10 oz
- 2 tablespoons grass-fed butter
- Salt and pepper, to taste

For the Bacon-Wrapped Green Beans:

- 8-10 fresh green beans
- 4 slices of bacon
- Salt and pepper, to taste

How To Cook

For the New York Steak:

- Preheat your oven to 400°F (200°C).
- Season the New York steak generously with salt and pepper on both sides.
- Heat an oven-safe skillet over high heat and add the grass-fed butter.
- Once the butter is melted and foamy, add the New York steak to the skillet.
- Sear the steak for 2-3 minutes on each side, or until a crust forms.
- Transfer the skillet with the steak to the preheated oven and cook for an additional 5-10 minutes, or until the desired internal temperature is reached (medium-rare is around 130°F (54°C)).
- Remove the skillet from the oven and let the steak rest for a few minutes before slicing.

For the Bacon-Wrapped Green Beans:

- Preheat your oven to 400°F (200°C).
- Rinse and trim the ends of the green beans.
- Wrap each green bean with a slice of bacon and secure with a toothpick.
- Place the bacon-wrapped green beans on a baking sheet lined with parchment paper.
- Season with salt and pepper to taste.
- Bake in the preheated oven for 12-15 minutes, or until the bacon is crispy and the green beans are tender.
- Remove from the oven and let cool for a few minutes before serving.
- To Serve:
- Slice the New York steak against the grain into thin slices.
- Arrange the steak slices on a plate along with the bacon-wrapped green beans.
- Drizzle any juices from the skillet over the steak for added flavor. Enjoy!

OPTIMUM BEEF SCRAMBLE

What You Need

- 1/2 lb ground beef
- 4 large eggs
- 1 tablespoon butter or cooking oil
- 1/4 cup nutritional yeast
- 1/2 red bell pepper, diced
- 1/2 green bell pepper, diced
- Salt and pepper to taste
- 1 avocado, diced

How To Cook

- Heat a skillet over medium-high heat and add the butter or cooking oil.
- Add the ground beef to the skillet and cook until browned and cooked through. Break up the beef into smaller pieces as it cooks.
- Add the diced red and green bell peppers to the skillet and cook for a few minutes until they are slightly softened.
- Crack the eggs into the skillet with the beef and peppers. Season with salt and pepper to taste.
- Stir the eggs, beef, and peppers together in the skillet and cook until the eggs are fully cooked to your liking.
- Remove the skillet from the heat and stir in the nutritional yeast.
- Transfer the beef scramble to serving plates and top with diced avocado.
- Serve hot and enjoy your high-fat keto beef scramble with nutritional yeast, peppers, and avocado!
- Note: You can adjust the seasoning and add other keto-friendly ingredients such as cheese or herbs to suit your taste preferences. Nutritional values may vary depending on the specific ingredients and quantities used.

OPTIMUM BREAKFAST BOWL

What You Need

- 4 slices of bacon
- 4 breakfast sausage links
- 4 large eggs
- 1/4 cup shredded cheddar cheese
- 1 tablespoon unfortified nutritional yeast
- Salt and pepper, to taste
- Optional toppings: sliced avocado, chopped tomatoes, hot sauce

How To Cook

- In a large skillet, cook the bacon over medium heat until crispy. Remove from the pan and set aside.
- In the same skillet, cook the breakfast sausage until browned and cooked through. Remove from the pan and set aside.
- Crack the eggs into the skillet and cook to your desired doneness.
- Top your bowl with shredded cheddar cheese, and season with salt and pepper, to taste.
- Sprinkle the nutritional yeast seasoning mixture over the entire dish.
- If desired, add additional toppings such as sliced avocado, cayenne pepper, or hot sauce.
- Serve immediately and enjoy!

PAN FRIED SALMON with ASPARAGUS

What You Need

- 2 salmon filets
- Salt and black pepper, to taste
- 1 tbsp olive oil
- 1 lb asparagus, trimmed
- 2 cloves garlic, minced
- 2 tbsp butter

How To Cook

- Season the salmon filets with salt and black pepper on both sides.
- Heat a large skillet over medium-high heat and add the olive oil.
- Add the salmon filets to the skillet and cook for 3-4 minutes on each side, until browned and cooked through.
- Once the salmon filets are cooked, remove them from the skillet and set them aside on a plate.
- In the same skillet, add the trimmed asparagus and minced garlic. Cook for 3-4 minutes until the asparagus is tender but still slightly crisp.
- Add the butter to the skillet and stir until it has melted and coats the asparagus.
- Season the asparagus with salt and black pepper to taste.
- Once the asparagus is cooked, remove it from the skillet and serve alongside the salmon filets.
- Optional: You can squeeze some lemon juice over the salmon filets and asparagus for added flavor.

PAN SEARED RIBEYE with BACON ASPARAGUS

What You Need

For the Pan-Seared Ribeye:

- 1 ribeye steak (about 1 lb)
- 2 tbsp butter
- Salt and pepper to taste
- Fresh thyme or rosemary for garnish (optional)

For the Bacon-Wrapped Asparagus:

- 1 lb asparagus spears, trimmed
- 8-10 slices of bacon
- Salt and pepper to taste
- Olive oil for drizzling

How To Cook

- Prepare the Bacon-Wrapped Asparagus:
- Preheat your oven to 400°F (200°C).
- Wrap each asparagus spear with a slice of bacon, starting at the base and wrapping it tightly towards the tip.
- Place the bacon-wrapped asparagus on a baking sheet lined with foil.
- Drizzle with olive oil and season with salt and pepper to taste.
- Bake in the preheated oven for 12-15 minutes, or until the bacon is crispy and the asparagus is tender. Remove from the oven and set aside.
- Prepare the Pan-Seared Ribeye:
- Pat dry the ribeye steak with paper towels to remove excess moisture, which helps with searing.
- Season both sides of the ribeye steak generously with salt and pepper.
- In a cast iron skillet or a heavy-bottomed skillet over high heat, melt the butter.
- Add the ribeye steak to the hot skillet and sear for 3-4 minutes per side for medium-rare, or until your desired level of doneness is reached.
- Use tongs to flip the steak only once during cooking to get a good sear.
- Remove the ribeye steak from the skillet and let it rest for a few minutes before slicing. This helps to retain the juices and keep the steak juicy and tender.

PANCAKES and SAUSAGE with BACON

What You Need

- 2 large eggs
- 2 oz cream cheese, softened
- 2 tbsp coconut flour
- 2 tbsp almond flour
- 2 tbsp heavy cream
- 1 tbsp melted butter
- 1/2 tsp baking powder
- 1/2 tsp vanilla extract
- 1/4 tsp salt
- 2 tbsp nutritional yeast
- Cooking oil or butter for frying
- 2 sausage links
- 4 slices of bacon

How To Cook

- In a mixing bowl, combine the eggs, cream cheese, coconut flour, almond flour, heavy cream, melted butter, baking powder, vanilla extract, salt, and nutritional yeast. Whisk until smooth and well combined.
- Heat a non-stick skillet or griddle over medium heat and grease with cooking oil or butter.
- Scoop 1/4 cup of the pancake batter onto the hot skillet and spread it out into a circle using the back of a spoon. Cook for 2-3 minutes on each side until bubbles form on the surface and the edges are slightly crispy. Remove from the skillet and set aside. Repeat with the remaining batter to make more pancakes.
- In a separate skillet, cook the sausage links and bacon slices over medium heat until cooked through. Remove from the skillet and set aside.

PAN SEARED SALMON and GREEN BEANS

What You Need

- 2 salmon filets, skin-on
- Salt and pepper
- 1 tbsp olive oil
- 2 cloves garlic, minced
- 1 tbsp chopped fresh rosemary
- 1 tbsp chopped fresh thyme
- 1 lb green beans, trimmed
- 1 tbsp butter
- Lemon wedges for serving

How To Cook

- Pat the salmon filets dry with a paper towel and season with salt and pepper on both sides.
- Heat the olive oil in a large skillet over medium-high heat.
- Add the salmon filets to the skillet, skin-side down, and cook for 4-5 minutes, until the skin is crispy.
- Flip the salmon filets and add the minced garlic, rosemary, and thyme to the skillet. Cook for another 4-5 minutes, until the salmon is cooked through.
- While the salmon is cooking, blanch the green beans in a pot of boiling salted water for 2-3 minutes, until they are tender but still crisp.
- Drain the green beans and toss them in the skillet with the butter and any remaining herbs and garlic.
- Serve the salmon and green beans hot, with lemon wedges on the side.
- This pan-seared salmon and green beans recipe is a delicious and healthy meal that is quick and easy to make. Enjoy!

PARMESAN-CRUSTED PORK CHOPS with ROASTED ASPARAGUS

What You Need

For the pork chops:

- 4 boneless pork chops
- 1/2 cup grated Parmesan cheese
- 1/2 cup almond flour
- 1/2 tsp garlic powder
- 1/2 tsp dried basil
- 1/2 tsp dried oregano
- Salt and pepper, to taste
- 2 tbsp olive oil

For the roasted asparagus:

- 1 lb asparagus, trimmed
- 2 tbsp olive oil
- Salt and pepper, to taste

How To Cook

For the pork chops:

- Preheat your oven to 400°F (200°C).
- In a shallow bowl, mix together the grated Parmesan cheese, almond flour, garlic powder, dried basil, dried oregano, salt, and pepper.
- Dip each pork chop in the Parmesan mixture, pressing the mixture onto the chops to make sure they are fully coated.
- In a large skillet, heat 2 tablespoons of olive oil over medium-high heat. Once hot, add the pork chops to the skillet.
- Cook the pork chops for 3-4 minutes on each side, until the coating is crispy and golden brown.
- Transfer the pork chops to a baking sheet lined with parchment paper.
- Bake in the preheated oven for 10-12 minutes, or until the pork chops are cooked through.

For the roasted asparagus:

- Arrange the trimmed asparagus on a baking sheet lined with parchment paper.
- Drizzle 2 tablespoons of olive oil over the asparagus and sprinkle with salt and pepper to taste.
- Roast the asparagus in the preheated oven for 10-15 minutes, or until tender and slightly crispy. Enjoy!

POACHED EGGS with SAUSAGE

What You Need

- 4 large eggs
- 4 sausages of your choice
- 2 tablespoons butter
- Salt and black pepper to taste
- Chopped fresh parsley for garnish (optional)

How To Cook

- Bring a pot of water to a gentle simmer over medium-low heat. Avoid boiling the water as it can cause the eggs to break apart.
- While the water is heating, cook the sausages in a skillet over medium heat until they are cooked through and nicely browned. Remove the sausages from the skillet and set them aside.
- Crack one egg into a small bowl or ramekin. Repeat with the remaining eggs.
- Once the water is simmering, carefully slide the eggs, one at a time, into the simmering water. Cook for about 3-4 minutes for a runny yolk or 5-6 minutes for a slightly firmer yolk.
- Using a slotted spoon, carefully remove the poached eggs from the water and place them on a paper towel-lined plate to drain any excess water.
- In the same skillet used to cook the sausages, melt the butter over medium heat.
- Add the poached eggs to the skillet with the melted butter and gently swirl the butter around the eggs to coat them.
- Season the eggs with salt and black pepper to taste.
- Place one sausage on each plate, and carefully transfer a poached egg on top of each sausage.
- Enjoy!

PORK CHOPS with EGGS and AVOCADO

What You Need

- 1 thick-cut pork chops
- Salt and pepper to taste
- Cooking oil or butter for cooking
- 4 large eggs
- 1 ripe avocado, sliced
- 1 tablespoon nutritional yeast

How To Cook

- Season the pork chop generously with salt and pepper on both sides.
- Heat a skillet over medium-high heat and add cooking oil or butter.
- Add the pork chops to the skillet and cook for about 4-5 minutes per side, or until they reach an internal temperature of 145°F (63°C) for medium doneness. Adjust cooking time based on the thickness of the pork chops and your desired level of doneness.
- Once the pork chop is cooked, transfer it to a plate and let it rest for a few minutes.
- In the same skillet, add more cooking oil or butter if needed. Crack the eggs into the skillet and cook to your desired level of doneness. You can fry them sunny-side up, over easy, or however you prefer.
- While the eggs are cooking, slice the ripe avocado.
- Once the eggs are cooked, carefully transfer them to the same plate as the pork chop.
- Sprinkle the nutritional yeast over the pork chop, eggs, and avocado slices.
- Serve hot and enjoy your pork chop with eggs, avocado, and nutritional yeast!

PORK CHOPS with ZUCCHINI

What You Need

- 1 pork chop (approx 6 oz)
- Salt and pepper
- 1 tbsp olive oil
- 1 small zucchini, sliced
- 1 clove garlic, minced
- 1 tbsp butter
- 1 tbsp grated Parmesan cheese
- 1 tablespoon nutritional yeast

How To Cook

- Preheat the oven to 375°F.
- Season the pork chop with salt and pepper on both sides.
- In a large skillet, heat the olive oil over medium-high heat. Once hot, add the pork chop and cook for 3-4 minutes on each side, or until browned.
- Transfer the pork chop to a baking dish and bake in the oven for 10-12 minutes, or until fully cooked.
- While the pork chop is baking, add the sliced zucchini to the same skillet used for the pork. Cook over medium heat for 3-4 minutes, or until lightly browned.
- Add the minced garlic and cook for an additional 30 seconds, or until fragrant.
- Remove the skillet from the heat and stir in the butter until melted.
- Once the pork chop is done, remove it from the oven and let it rest for a few minutes.
- Spoon the zucchini and garlic mixture over the pork chop, and sprinkle with grated Parmesan cheese and nutritional yeast. Enjoy!

PROSCIUTTO WRAPPED SEA SCALLOPS with BROCCOLI

What You Need

For the Prosciutto-Wrapped Scallops:

- 12 large scallops, patted dry
- 6 thin slices of prosciutto, cut in half lengthwise
- 2 tbsp butter, melted
- Salt and pepper to taste
- Lemon wedges for serving (optional)

For the Broccoli:

- 1 lb broccoli florets
- 2 tbsp olive oil
- 2 cloves garlic, minced
- Salt and pepper to taste

How To Cook

- Prepare the Prosciutto-Wrapped Scallops:
- Preheat your oven to 400°F (200°C) and line a baking sheet with parchment paper.
- Wrap each scallop with half a slice of prosciutto, securing it with a toothpick if needed
- Place the prosciutto-wrapped scallops on the prepared baking sheet.
- Brush the melted butter over the scallops and season with salt and pepper to taste.
- Bake in the preheated oven for 12-15 minutes, or until the scallops are cooked through and the prosciutto is crispy. Remove from the oven and set aside.
- Prepare the Broccoli:
- While the scallops are baking, prepare the broccoli
- In a large bowl, toss the broccoli florets with olive oil, minced garlic, salt, and pepper.
- Spread the seasoned broccoli florets in a single layer on a baking sheet lined with parchment paper.
- Roast in the oven at 400°F (200°C) for 10-12 minutes, or until the broccoli is tender and lightly browned
- Enjoy!

RIBEYE ASPARAGUS ARUGULA

What You Need

For the ribeye steak:

- 1 ribeye steak (about 1 inch thick)
- Salt and pepper, to taste
- 2 tablespoons grass-fed butter

For the asparagus:

- 1 bunch of asparagus, woody ends trimmed
- 2 tablespoons olive oil
- Salt and pepper, to taste

For the arugula salad:

- 4 cups fresh arugula
- 2 tablespoons extra-virgin olive oil
- 1 tablespoon vinegar (such as balsamic or red wine vinegar)
- Salt and pepper, to taste

How To Cook

- Let the ribeye steak come to room temperature for about 30 minutes before cooking. This helps to ensure even cooking.
- Preheat your oven to 400°F (200°C). Place the trimmed asparagus on a baking sheet and drizzle with olive oil. Season with salt and pepper, then toss to coat. Roast in the preheated oven for 10-12 minutes, until tender and slightly charred.
- While the asparagus is roasting, season the ribeye steak generously with salt and pepper on both sides.
- Heat a cast-iron skillet or oven-safe skillet over medium-high heat. Add the grass-fed butter to the skillet and let it melt. Once the butter is foamy, add the ribeye steak to the skillet and sear for about 3-4 minutes per side, until a crust forms and the internal temperature reaches your desired level of doneness (130°F for medium-rare, 135°F for medium).
- Transfer the ribeye steak to a cutting board and let it rest for a few minutes before slicing it against the grain.
- In a small bowl, whisk together the extra-virgin olive oil, vinegar, salt, and pepper to make the vinaigrette for the arugula salad.
- In a large bowl, toss the arugula with the vinaigrette until well coated. Enjoy!

RIBEYE EGGS ASPARAGUS AVOCADO

What You Need

- 1 ribeye steak
- 2 eggs
- Asparagus spears
- 2 tablespoons grass-fed butter
- 1 tablespoon olive oil
- Salt and pepper to taste
- 1 tablespoon nutritional yeast

How To Cook

Prepare the Ribeye Steak:

- Season the ribeye steak with salt and pepper on both sides.
- Heat a skillet over medium-high heat and add 1 tablespoon of olive oil.
- Once the oil is hot, add the ribeye steak to the skillet and cook for about 3-4 minutes per side for medium-rare or until your desired level of doneness.
- Remove the ribeye steak from the skillet and let it rest for a few minutes before slicing it.

Cook the Asparagus:

- Rinse the asparagus spears and trim off the tough ends.
- In the same skillet used to cook the ribeye steak, add 1 tablespoon of grass-fed butter over medium heat.
- Add the asparagus spears to the skillet and cook for about 4-5 minutes, stirring occasionally, until they are tender and slightly charred.
- Season the asparagus with salt and pepper to taste.

Cook the Eggs:

- In a separate non-stick skillet, melt 1 tablespoon of grass-fed butter over medium heat.
- Crack the eggs into the skillet and cook until the whites are set but the yolks are still slightly runny, or to your desired level of doneness.
- Season the eggs with salt and pepper to taste.
- Add the nutritional yeast
- Assemble the Meal:
- Place the cooked ribeye steak on a plate.
- Arrange the cooked asparagus spears alongside the steak.
- Top the ribeye steak with the fried eggs.
- Drizzle some extra virgin olive oil over the steak, eggs, and asparagus. Enjoy!

RIBEYE STEAK with CREAMED SPINACH and MUSHROOM

What You Need

- 1 ribeye steak (about 1 pound)
- 2 tablespoons of olive oil
- 2 cloves of garlic, minced
- Salt and pepper
- 1 cup of sliced mushrooms
- 2 cups of fresh spinach
- 1/2 cup of heavy cream
- 2 tablespoons of butter

How To Cook

- Take the ribeye steak out of the fridge and let it sit at room temperature for about 30 minutes before cooking. This will help it cook more evenly.
- In a skillet over medium heat, add 1 tablespoon of olive oil and minced garlic. Sauté for 1-2 minutes until fragrant.
- Add sliced mushrooms to the skillet and cook for about 5-7 minutes until they are browned and tender. Season with salt and pepper to taste.
- Remove the mushrooms from the skillet and set aside. Add another tablespoon of olive oil to the skillet.
- Season the ribeye steak generously with salt and pepper on both sides.
- Place the steak in the skillet and cook for about 3-4 minutes on each side for medium-rare, or until the desired level of doneness is reached. Use tongs to flip the steak to avoid piercing it with a fork.
- Remove the steak from the skillet and let it rest on a cutting board for 5-10 minutes.
- While the steak is resting, add butter to the skillet and melt over medium heat. Add fresh spinach and cook for about 2-3 minutes until wilted.
- Pour in heavy cream and stir until the sauce thickens. Add the sautéed mushrooms to the skillet and stir to combine.
- Slice the steak against the grain and serve with the creamed spinach and mushroom sauce.

SAUSAGE and EGGS with HAMBURGER

What You Need

For the Hamburger Patty

- 1/2 lb ground beef
- 1/4 tsp salt
- 1/4 tsp black pepper
- 1/4 tsp garlic powder
- 1/4 tsp onion powder
- 1/4 tsp paprika
- 1/4 tsp dried oregano
- 1/4 tsp dried basil
- 1/4 tsp red pepper flakes (optional)
- 2 tbsp butter or ghee for cooking

For the Sausage and Eggs:

- 4 sausage links
- 4 large eggs
- 2 tbsp butter or ghee
- Salt and pepper to tast

How To Cook

- Prepare the Hamburger Patty:
- In a mixing bowl, combine the ground beef with salt, pepper, garlic powder, onion powder, paprika, dried oregano, dried basil, and red pepper flakes (if using).
- Mix well with your hands or a fork until the spices are evenly distributed.
- Divide the seasoned ground beef into 2 portions and shape each portion into a patty.
- In a skillet over medium-high heat, melt the butter or ghee.
- Add the hamburger patties to the hot skillet and cook for 3-4 minutes per side, or until cooked to your desired level of doneness.
- Remove the hamburger patties from the skillet and set them aside.
- Prepare the Sausage and Eggs:
- In the same skillet used for the hamburger patties, add the sausage links.
- Cook the sausage links over medium heat for 4-5 minutes per side, or until cooked through and nicely browned.
- Remove the cooked sausage links from the skillet and set them aside.
- In the same skillet, melt the butter or ghee over medium heat.
- Crack the eggs into the skillet and season them with salt and pepper to taste.
- Cook the eggs to your desired level of doneness, either sunny-side up, over easy, or over hard. Enjoy!

SAUSAGE PATTY SANDWICHES

What You Need

- 4 sausage patties (choose a brand that is low in carbs and high in fat)
- 4 slices of bacon
- 4 slices of cheese (cheddar, Swiss, or any cheese of your choice)
- 4 large eggs
- 1 ripe avocado, sliced
- Lettuce leaves (optional, for serving)
- Tomato slices (optional, for serving)
- Salt and pepper to taste
- Cooking oil or butter for frying

How To Cook

- Cook the sausage patties and bacon according to package instructions or your preferred method. If using a stovetop skillet, cook the sausage patties and bacon over medium heat until they are cooked through and crispy. Drain excess grease on paper towels, if necessary.
- Place a slice of cheese on top of each sausage patty while they are still hot, allowing the cheese to melt slightly.
- In a separate skillet, cook the eggs to your desired level of doneness (fried, over-easy, etc.) using cooking oil or butter. Season with salt and pepper to taste.
- Assemble the sandwich by placing a sausage patty with melted cheese on the bottom, followed by a slice of bacon, a cooked egg, and slices of avocado on top.
- If desired, add lettuce leaves and tomato slices to the sandwich.
- Serve the sausage patties sandwich with cheese, bacon, egg, and avocado and enjoy!

SEAFOOD SALAD

What You Need

- 1 lb cooked shrimp, peeled and deveined
- 1 lb cooked lump crabmeat
- 1/2 cup diced celery
- 1/2 cup diced red bell pepper
- 1/4 cup chopped fresh parsley
- 1/4 cup mayonnaise
- 1 tbsp Dijon mustard
- 1 tbsp fresh lemon juice
- 1 tsp Old Bay seasoning
- Salt and pepper, to taste
- Lettuce leaves, for serving

How To Cook

- In a large bowl, combine the cooked shrimp, crabmeat, celery, red bell pepper, and parsley.
- In a small bowl, whisk together the mayonnaise, Dijon mustard, lemon juice, and Old Bay seasoning.
- Pour the dressing over the seafood mixture and toss to coat.
- Season with salt and pepper, to taste.
- Chill the seafood salad in the refrigerator for at least 30 minutes before serving.
- Serve the seafood salad on a bed of lettuce leaves.

SHRIMP and BURGER PATTY with ASPARAGUS

What You Need

For the Burger Patty:
- 4 oz ground beef (preferably grass-fed)
- 1/4 teaspoon salt
- 1/4 teaspoon black pepper
- 1 tablespoon grass-fed butter, melted

For the Shrimp:
- 6 oz raw shrimp, peeled and deveined
- 1 tablespoon grass-fed butter
- 1 small clove garlic, minced
- 1/4 teaspoon paprika
- Salt and pepper, to taste

For the Asparagus:
- 8-10 stalks of asparagus
- 1 tablespoon avocado oil or coconut oil
- Salt and pepper, to taste

How To Cook

- Preheat your oven to 375°F (190°C).
- In a bowl, combine the ground beef, salt, and black pepper. Form the mixture into a patty.
- Heat a skillet over medium-high heat and add the melted grass-fed butter.
- Place the burger patty in the skillet and cook for about 3-4 minutes per side, or until it reaches your desired level of doneness. Remove from the skillet and set aside.
- In the same skillet, add the raw shrimp, minced garlic, paprika, salt, and pepper. Cook for about 2-3 minutes per side, or until the shrimp turn pink and are cooked through. Remove from the skillet and set aside.
- Place the asparagus stalks on a baking sheet lined with parchment paper.
- Drizzle the avocado oil or coconut oil over the asparagus and season with salt and pepper to taste.
- Roast the asparagus in the preheated oven for 10-12 minutes, or until they are tender but still slightly crisp.
- To serve, place the cooked burger patty and shrimp on a plate, along with the roasted asparagus. Enjoy!

SPINACH and FETA STUFFED CHICKEN BREAST

What You Need

- 2 boneless, skinless chicken breasts
- Salt and pepper to taste
- 1/2 cup chopped fresh spinach
- 1/4 cup crumbled feta cheese
- 1 clove garlic, minced
- 1 tbsp olive oil
- 1 tbsp butter

How To Cook

- Preheat the oven to 375°F (190°C).
- Use a sharp knife to make a horizontal cut in the thickest part of each chicken breast, being careful not to cut all the way through.
- Open up each chicken breast and season the inside with salt and pepper.
- In a small bowl, mix together the chopped spinach, feta cheese, and minced garlic.
- Stuff the spinach and feta mixture into the pocket of each chicken breast, packing it in tightly.
- Use toothpicks to secure the opening of each chicken breast.
- Heat the olive oil and butter in an oven-safe skillet over medium-high heat.
- Sear the stuffed chicken breasts for 2-3 minutes on each side, or until golden brown.
- Transfer the skillet to the preheated oven and bake for 20-25 minutes, or until the chicken is cooked through and the juices run clear.
- Remove the toothpicks from the chicken and serve hot.
- Enjoy your Spinach and Feta Stuffed Chicken Breast!

SPINACH and MUSHROOM OMELET with CHEESEBURGER

What You Need

For the cheeseburger patty:
- 1/4 lb ground beef
- 1 tablespoon of nutritional yeast
- 1/4 tsp salt
- 1/4 tsp black pepper
- 1/4 tsp garlic powder
- 1/4 tsp onion powder
- 1/4 cup shredded cheese

For the omelet:
3 large eggs
1 tablespoon butter
1 cup spinach, chopped
1/2 cup mushrooms, sliced
1/4 cup shredded cheese
Salt and black pepper to taste

How To Cook

- For the cheeseburger patty:
- In a bowl, combine the ground beef, salt, black pepper, garlic powder, and onion powder. Mix well.
- Form the seasoned ground beef into a patty shape and press a small amount of shredded cheese into the center of the patty.
- Cook the cheeseburger patty in a skillet or on a grill over medium-high heat until it reaches your desired level of doneness, typically about 3-4 minutes per side.
- Once cooked, remove the cheeseburger patty from the skillet or grill and set aside.
- For the omelet:
- In a bowl, beat the eggs with a pinch of salt and black pepper.
- Heat a non-stick skillet over medium heat and melt the butter or coconut oil.
- Add the chopped spinach and sliced mushrooms to the skillet and cook until they start to soften, about 2-3 minutes.
- Pour the beaten eggs over the spinach and mushrooms in the skillet, and cook until the edges are set and the center is slightly runny, about 3-4 minutes.
- Sprinkle the shredded cheese and nutritional yeast evenly over one half of the omelet.
- Carefully place the cheeseburger patty on top of the cheese on the omelet.
- Fold the other half of the omelet over the cheeseburger patty, using a spatula to help if needed.
- Cook for another 1-2 minutes until the cheese is melted and the omelet is cooked through. Enjoy!

STEAK SALAD with AVOCADO

What You Need

- 1 lb flank steak
- Salt and pepper, to taste
- 4 cups mixed greens
- 1 avocado, sliced
- 1/4 cup crumbled blue cheese
- 1/4 cup chopped red onion
- 2 tablespoons olive oil
- 2 tablespoons red wine vinegar
- 1 clove garlic, minced

How To Cook

- Preheat the grill or grill pan to high heat.
- Season the flank steak with salt and pepper to taste.
- Grill the steak for 5-6 minutes per side for medium-rare, or until cooked to your desired level of doneness.
- Let the steak rest for a few minutes, then slice it thinly against the grain.
- In a large bowl, combine the mixed greens, sliced avocado, crumbled blue cheese, and chopped red onion.
- In a small bowl, whisk together the olive oil, red wine vinegar, and minced garlic. Season with salt and pepper to taste.
- Drizzle the dressing over the salad and toss to coat.
- Top the salad with the sliced steak.
- Serve immediately.
- Emjoy!

STUFFED BELL PEPPERS

What You Need

- 4 large bell peppers (any color)
- 1 pound ground beef or sausage (choose a higher fat content)
- 1/2 cup diced onion
- 2 cloves garlic, minced
- 1/2 cup diced tomatoes
- 1/2 cup shredded mozzarella cheese
- 1/4 cup grated parmesan cheese
- 2 tablespoons tomato paste
- 1 tablespoon olive oil
- 1 teaspoon Italian seasoning
- 1/2 teaspoon salt
- 1/4 teaspoon black pepper
- Fresh basil leaves for garnish (optional)

How To Cook

- Preheat your oven to 375°F (190°C). Line a baking dish with foil or parchment paper for easy cleanup.
- Cut the tops off the bell peppers and remove the seeds and membranes from the inside. Rinse the bell peppers and place them in the prepared baking dish.
- In a large skillet, heat the olive oil over medium heat. Add the diced onion and minced garlic, and sauté until softened, about 3-4 minutes.
- Add the ground beef or sausage to the skillet, and cook until browned, breaking it up with a spoon as it cooks. Drain any excess grease if needed.
- Stir in the diced tomatoes, tomato paste, Italian seasoning, salt, and black pepper. Cook for another 2-3 minutes to combine the flavors.
- Remove the skillet from heat, and stir in the shredded mozzarella cheese and grated parmesan cheese.
- Spoon the meat and cheese mixture into the hollowed-out bell peppers, packing it tightly.
- Bake the stuffed bell peppers in the preheated oven for 25-30 minutes, or until the peppers are tender and the cheese is melted and bubbly.
- Enjoy your stuffed bell peppers!

TACO SALAD

What You Need

- 1 lb ground beef
- 1 tbsp olive oil
- 1 tbsp chili powder
- 1 tsp ground cumin
- 1 tsp garlic powder
- 1/2 tsp onion powder
- Salt and pepper to taste
- 4 cups chopped romaine lettuce
- 1 avocado, diced
- 1/2 cup shredded cheddar cheese
- 1/4 cup diced red onion
- 1/4 cup chopped fresh cilantro
- 1/4 cup sour cream
- 2 tbsp salsa
- 1 lime, cut into wedges

How To Cook

- Heat olive oil in a large skillet over medium-high heat.
- Add the ground beef to the skillet and cook until browned and fully cooked, breaking it up with a spatula as it cooks.
- Stir in chili powder, ground cumin, garlic powder, onion powder, salt, and pepper. Cook for an additional 1-2 minutes until the spices are fragrant.
- In a large bowl, toss together chopped romaine lettuce, diced avocado, shredded cheddar cheese, diced red onion, and chopped cilantro.
- Divide the lettuce mixture into serving bowls or plates.
- Spoon the cooked ground beef over the lettuce mixture.
- Top the salad with sour cream, salsa, and lime wedges.
- Serve and enjoy!

THE OPTIMUM BREAKFAST

What You Need

- 4 eggs
- 3 slices of bacon
- 1 slice of grass-fed cheese (your preferred type)
- 1 hamburger patty
- 1 ripe avocado
- Grass-fed butter for cooking (as needed)
- 1 tablespoon unfortified nutritional yeast
- Ancient sea salt (to taste)
- Pepper (to taste)
- Garlic powder (to taste)
- Olive oil (for drizzling)

How To Cook

- Cook the bacon slices in a skillet over medium heat until crispy. Remove from the skillet and set aside on paper towels to drain excess grease.
- In the same skillet, cook the hamburger patty according to your desired level of doneness, using grass-fed butter for cooking as needed. Set aside.
- In a separate skillet, melt some grass-fed butter over medium heat.
- Crack the eggs into the skillet with the melted butter and cook until the whites are set but the yolks are still slightly runny, basting the eggs with the melted butter for added flavor. Season the eggs with ancient sea salt, pepper, and garlic powder to taste.
- While the eggs are cooking, cut the avocado in half, remove the pit, and scoop out the flesh. Slice the avocado into thin pieces.
- Once the eggs are cooked, carefully flip them over to cook for an additional minute if you prefer them fully cooked.
- Place the cooked hamburger patty on a plate. Top with a slice of grass-fed cheese to melt.
- Place the cooked bacon slices on top of the cheese.
- Arrange the sliced avocado on the plate next to the hamburger patty.
- Carefully place the cooked eggs on top of the avocado slices.
- In a small bowl, combine the unfortified nutritional yeast with ancient sea salt, pepper, and garlic powder to taste.
- Drizzle olive oil over the hamburger patty, eggs, and avocado for added flavor.
- Sprinkle the yeast and enjoy!

TOMATO SOUP with GRILLED CHEESE BITES

What You Need

For the tomato soup:

- 1 tbsp olive oil
- 1/2 onion, diced
- 2 cloves garlic, minced
- 28 oz can of crushed tomatoes
- 1 cup chicken broth
- 1/2 cup heavy cream
- 1/2 tsp dried basil
- 1/2 tsp dried oregano
- Salt and pepper, to taste

For the grilled cheese bites:

- 2 slices of Keto bread, toasted
- 1 oz cheddar cheese, shredded
- 1 oz mozzarella cheese, shredded
- 1 tbsp butter

How To Cook

For the tomato soup:

- Heat the olive oil in a pot over medium heat. Add the diced onion and minced garlic, and sauté until the onion is translucent and the garlic is fragrant.
- Add the crushed tomatoes, chicken broth, dried basil, dried oregano, salt, and pepper to the pot. Stir to combine.
- Bring the soup to a simmer and let it cook for 15-20 minutes.
- Add the heavy cream to the pot and stir to combine.
- Use an immersion blender to puree the soup until smooth. If you don't have an immersion blender, you can transfer the soup to a blender and puree it in batches.
- Adjust the seasoning to taste.

For the grilled cheese bites:

- Preheat a non-stick skillet over medium heat.
- Mix together the shredded cheddar cheese and shredded mozzarella cheese in a small bowl.
- Spread 1 tablespoon of butter on one side of each slice of toasted Keto bread.
- Sprinkle the cheese mixture on the unbuttered side of one slice of bread and top it with the other slice of bread, buttered side up.
- Place the sandwich in the skillet and cook until the cheese is melted and the bread is crispy, about 2-3 minutes per side. Serve and Enjoy!

TURKEY BURGER with ARUGULA

What You Need

For Turkey Cheese Burgers:
- 1 pound ground turkey
- 1/2 cup grated cheddar cheese
- 1/4 cup mayonnaise
- 2 cloves garlic, minced
- 1 tablespoon Worcestershire sauce
- 1/2 teaspoon salt
- 1/4 teaspoon black pepper
- 4 slices of cheddar cheese (optional)
- 4 lettuce leaves (for wrapping the burgers)

For Arugula Salad:
- 4 cups arugula
- 1/4 cup olive oil
- 2 tablespoons lemon juice
- Salt and pepper to taste

How To Cook

- In a mixing bowl, combine ground turkey, grated cheddar cheese, mayonnaise, minced garlic, Worcestershire sauce, salt, and black pepper. Mix well to combine.
- Shape the mixture into 2 burger patties.
- Heat a grill or a pan over medium-high heat. Cook the turkey burger patties for about 5-6 minutes per side, or until they are cooked through and have an internal temperature of 165°F (75°C).
- Optional: Top each burger patty with a slice of cheddar cheese during the last minute of cooking and let it melt.
- While the burgers are cooking, prepare the arugula salad. In a large mixing bowl, whisk together olive oil, lemon juice, salt, and pepper to make the dressing. Add arugula to the bowl and toss to coat the leaves with the dressing.

TURKEY MEATLOAF with GREEN BEANS

What You Need

For the turkey meatloaf:

- 2 pounds ground turkey
- 1 cup almond flour
- 1/2 cup grated Parmesan cheese
- 2 eggs
- 1/2 cup chopped onion
- 1/2 cup chopped celery
- 1/2 cup chopped red bell pepper
- 1 tablespoon minced garlic
- 1 tablespoon Worcestershire sauce
- 1 tablespoon Dijon mustard
- 1 teaspoon dried thyme
- 1/2 teaspoon salt
- 1/2 teaspoon black pepper

For the green beans

- 1 pound fresh green beans, trimmed
- 2 tablespoons olive oil
- 2 tablespoon minced garlic
- Salt and pepper, to taste

How To Cook

- Preheat your oven to 375°F.
- In a large bowl, combine the ground turkey, almond flour, grated Parmesan cheese, eggs, chopped onion, chopped celery, chopped red bell pepper, minced garlic, Worcestershire sauce, Dijon mustard, dried thyme, salt, and black pepper. Mix until well combined.
- Transfer the turkey mixture to a 9x13 inch baking dish and shape it into a loaf.
- Bake the turkey meatloaf in the preheated oven for 50-60 minutes, or until the internal temperature reaches 165°F.
- While the meatloaf is baking, prepare the green beans. In a large skillet, heat the olive oil over medium-high heat. Add the minced garlic and sauté for 30 seconds, or until fragrant.
- Add the trimmed green beans to the skillet and sauté for 5-7 minutes, or until tender and lightly browned. Season with salt and pepper to taste.
- Plate and Enjoy!

TURKEY PATTY with EGGS BACON and AVOCADO

What You Need

- 1 lb ground turkey
- 1/2 tsp garlic powder
- 1/2 tsp onion powder
- 1/2 tsp smoked paprika
- 1 tablespoon nutritional yeast
- Salt and pepper, to taste
- 2 slices of bacon
- 2 eggs
- 1/2 avocado, sliced

How To Cook

For the turkey patty:

- In a mixing bowl, combine the ground turkey, garlic powder, onion powder, smoked paprika, nutritional yeast, salt, and pepper. Mix well to combine.
- Form the turkey mixture into 4 patties.
- Heat a skillet over medium heat and cook the patties for 4-5 minutes on each side, or until cooked through.

For the bacon and eggs:

- Cook the bacon in a skillet until crispy. Remove from the skillet and set aside.
- Crack the eggs into the same skillet and cook until the whites are set but the yolks are still runny.

To assemble:

- Place the cooked turkey patty on a plate.
- Top the patty with the bacon slices, fried eggs, and sliced avocado.
- This recipe is high in protein, healthy fats, and low in carbs, making it a perfect meal. Enjoy!

ZUCCHINI NOODLES in MEAT SAUCE

What You Need

- 2 medium zucchinis
- 1 pound ground beef
- 1 can (14 oz) diced tomatoes
- 1/2 onion, diced
- 2 garlic cloves, minced
- 2 tablespoons tomato paste
- 1 teaspoon dried basil
- 1 teaspoon dried oregano
- Salt and pepper to taste
- Olive oil for cooking

How To Cook

- Use a spiralizer to make zucchini noodles (zoodles) from the zucchinis. Set aside.
- Heat a large skillet over medium-high heat and add a drizzle of olive oil. Add the ground beef and cook until browned, breaking it up into smaller pieces as it cooks.
- Once the beef is browned, add the onion and garlic and sauté for 2-3 minutes until the onion is translucent.
- Add the diced tomatoes, tomato paste, dried basil, dried oregano, salt, and pepper to the skillet. Stir to combine.
- Bring the sauce to a simmer and let it cook for 5-10 minutes until it thickens.
- In a separate skillet, heat a drizzle of olive oil over medium-high heat. Add the zoodles and sauté for 2-3 minutes until tender.
- Serve the zoodles with the meat sauce on top. Enjoy!

BLACK and WHITE FAT BOMBS

What You Need

For the dark chocolate layer:

- 1/2 cup coconut oil, melted
- 1/4 cup unsweetened cocoa powder
- 1/4 cup powdered erythritol or stevia
- 1/2 tsp vanilla extract
- A pinch of salt

For the white vanilla layer:

- 1/2 cup coconut oil, melted
- 1/4 cup powdered erythritol or stevia (or any other sugar substitute to taste)
- 1 tsp vanilla extract
- A pinch of salt

How To Cook

- In a medium bowl, mix together the melted coconut oil, cocoa powder, powdered erythritol or stevia, vanilla extract, and a pinch of salt until well combined to make the dark chocolate layer.
- In a separate medium bowl, mix together the melted coconut oil, powdered erythritol or stevia, vanilla extract, and a pinch of salt until well combined to make the white vanilla layer.
- Line a silicone mold or small silicone ice cube tray with parchment paper.
- Spoon a small amount of the dark chocolate mixture into each mold cavity, filling it up to about 1/3 of the way.
- Spoon a small amount of the white vanilla mixture on top of the dark chocolate layer in each mold cavity, filling it up to about 2/3 of the way.
- Repeat with another layer of the dark chocolate mixture, filling it up to the top of each mold cavity.
- Use a toothpick or skewer to gently swirl the layers together to create a marbled effect.
- Place the mold or tray in the refrigerator or freezer to solidify for at least 30 minutes.
- Once fully solidified, pop the fat bombs out of the mold or tray and transfer them to an airtight container for storage. Enjoy!

CHOCOLATE AVOCADO MOUSSE

What You Need

- 2 ripe avocados
- 1/4 cup cocoa powder
- 1/4 cup coconut milk
- 1/4 cup powdered erythritol or stevia (or any other sugar substitute to taste)
- 1 tsp vanilla extract
- A pinch of salt
- Optional toppings: whipped cream, chopped nuts, or berries for garnish
- Instructions:

How To Cook

- Cut the avocados in half and remove the pits. Scoop out the flesh and place it in a blender or food processor.
- Add cocoa powder, coconut milk, powdered erythritol or stevia, vanilla extract, and a pinch of salt to the blender or food processor with the avocado.
- Blend on high speed until all the ingredients are well combined and the mixture is smooth and creamy.
- Taste and adjust sweetness as desired with more powdered erythritol or stevia.
- Transfer the chocolate avocado mousse to individual serving dishes or a larger bowl.
- Refrigerate for at least 1 hour to chill and set.
- Prior to serving, you can garnish with whipped cream, chopped nuts, or berries if desired.
- Enjoy your delicious homemade Chocolate Avocado Mousse as a satisfying and keto-friendly dessert!

FUDGY BROWNIES

What You Need

- 1/2 cup coconut flour
- 1/2 cup unsweetened cocoa powder
- 1/2 cup melted coconut oil
- 4 large eggs
- 1/2 cup powdered erythritol or stevia (or any other sugar substitute to taste)
- 1 tsp vanilla extract
- 1/2 tsp baking powder
- 1/4 tsp salt
- Optional: 1/2 cup chopped nuts, such as walnuts or pecans (optional)

How To Cook

- Preheat your oven to 350°F (175°C) and line an 8x8-inch baking pan with parchment paper.
- In a large bowl, whisk together the coconut flour, unsweetened cocoa powder, melted coconut oil, eggs, powdered erythritol or stevia, vanilla extract, baking powder, and salt until well combined.
- If using, stir in the chopped nuts into the brownie batter.
- Pour the brownie batter into the prepared baking pan and spread it out evenly.
- Bake in the preheated oven for 18-22 minutes, or until the edges are set and the center is slightly jiggly.
- Remove from the oven and let the brownies cool completely in the pan before cutting into squares.
- Enjoy these fudgy Keto Brownies as a decadent and low-carb dessert or snack!

KETO CHEESECAKE

What You Need

For the Crust:

- 1 1/2 cups almond flour
- 1/4 cup powdered erythritol or stevia
- 1/4 cup melted butter
- 1 tsp vanilla extract

For the Filling:

- 16 oz cream cheese, softened
- 2/3 cup powdered erythritol or stevia
- 2 large eggs
- 1 tsp vanilla extract

How To Cook

- Preheat your oven to 325°F (160°C). Grease a 9-inch springform pan and set aside.
- In a medium bowl, mix together almond flour, powdered erythritol or stevia, melted butter, and vanilla extract until well combined.
- Press the crust mixture firmly into the bottom of the prepared springform pan, forming an even layer.
- Bake the crust in the preheated oven for 10-12 minutes or until lightly golden. Remove from the oven and let it cool while you prepare the filling.

for the filling:

- In a large mixing bowl, beat the softened cream cheese until smooth using an electric mixer on low to medium speed.
- Add powdered erythritol or stevia, eggs, and vanilla extract to the cream cheese, and beat on low to medium speed until well combined and creamy.
- Scrape down the sides of the bowl with a spatula as needed to ensure all the ingredients are fully mixed.
- Pour the cream cheese filling over the cooled crust in the springform pan and smooth the top with a spatula.
- Tap the pan gently on the counter to remove any air bubbles.
- Bake the cheesecake in the preheated oven for 40-45 minutes or until the edges are set and the center is slightly jiggly.
- Turn off the oven, crack the oven door slightly, and let the cheesecake cool in the oven for 1 hour.
- After 1 hour, remove the cheesecake from the oven and let it cool completely at room temperature.
- Once fully cooled, cover the cheesecake with plastic wrap and refrigerate for at least 4 hours or overnight to allow it to set completely. Enjoy!

KETO CHOCOLATE ICE CREAM

What You Need

- 1 1/2 cups heavy cream
- 1/2 cup unsweetened almond milk or coconut milk
- 1/2 cup powdered erythritol or stevia
- 1/4 cup unsweetened cocoa powder
- 4 large egg yolks
- 2 tsp vanilla extract
- A pinch of salt

How To Cook

- In a saucepan, whisk together the heavy cream, almond milk or coconut milk, powdered erythritol or stevia, unsweetened cocoa powder, and a pinch of salt.
- Place the saucepan over medium heat and cook, stirring constantly, until the mixture reaches a temperature of about 170°F (77°C) and starts to steam, but do not let it boil.
- In a separate bowl, whisk the egg yolks until smooth.
- Slowly pour about 1/2 cup of the hot cream mixture into the egg yolks, whisking constantly to temper the yolks and prevent them from curdling.
- Pour the egg yolk mixture back into the saucepan with the remaining cream mixture, whisking constantly to combine.
- Cook the mixture over low heat, stirring constantly, until it thickens and coats the back of a spoon, about 5-7 minutes. Do not let it boil.
- Remove the saucepan from heat and stir in the vanilla extract.
- Let the ice cream mixture cool to room temperature, then cover and refrigerate for at least 4 hours or overnight to chill and fully develop the flavors.
- Once chilled, pour the ice cream mixture into an ice cream maker and churn according to the manufacturer's instructions.
- Transfer the churned ice cream to a lidded container and freeze for at least 4 hours or until firm. Enjoy

KETO COCONUT ALMOND FAT BOMBS

What You Need

- 1/2 cup coconut oil, melted
- 1/2 cup almond butter
- 1/4 cup unsweetened shredded coconut
- 1/4 cup powdered erythritol or stevia (or any other sugar substitute to taste)
- 1 tsp vanilla extract
- A pinch of salt
- Optional: sugar-free chocolate for drizzling (85% or higher cocoa content)

How To Cook

- In a medium bowl, mix together melted coconut oil, almond butter, shredded coconut, powdered erythritol or stevia, vanilla extract, and a pinch of salt until well combined.
- Spoon the mixture into silicone molds or small silicone ice cube trays.
- Place the molds or trays in the refrigerator or freezer to solidify for at least 30 minutes.
- If desired, you can melt some sugar-free chocolate in a microwave or double boiler and drizzle it over the solidified fat bombs for added flavor and decoration.
- Return the molds or trays to the refrigerator or freezer to set the chocolate, if using.
- Once fully solidified, pop the fat bombs out of the molds or trays and transfer them to an airtight container for storage.
- Enjoy these delicious Keto Coconut Almond Fat Bombs as a satisfying and convenient high-fat snack or dessert!
- Note: Store leftover fat bombs in an airtight container in the refrigerator or freezer, depending on your desired firmness. They can be stored for several weeks in the refrigerator or several months in the freezer.

KETO LEMON CHEESECAKE

What You Need

For the Crust:

- 1 cup almond flour
- 1/4 cup powdered erythritol or stevia
- 1/4 cup melted coconut oil

For the Filling:

- 16 oz cream cheese, softened
- 1/2 cup powdered erythritol or stevia
- 2 large eggs
- 1/4 cup fresh lemon juice
- 1 tbsp lemon zest
- 1 tsp vanilla extract

How To Cook

- Preheat your oven to 325°F (160°C) and line the bottom of a 9-inch springform pan with parchment paper.
- In a medium bowl, mix together almond flour, powdered erythritol or stevia, and melted coconut oil until well combined.
- Press the mixture evenly into the bottom of the prepared springform pan to form the crust.
- In a large bowl, beat the softened cream cheese and powdered erythritol or stevia with an electric mixer on low speed until smooth and creamy.
- Add in the eggs, one at a time, beating well after each addition.
- Mix in the fresh lemon juice, lemon zest, and vanilla extract until well combined.
- Pour the cream cheese filling over the crust in the springform pan.
- Tap the pan on the counter a few times to remove any air bubbles.
- Bake in the preheated oven for 40-45 minutes or until the edges are set and the center is slightly jiggly.
- Turn off the oven and crack the oven door open. Let the cheesecake cool in the oven for 1 hour.
- Remove the cheesecake from the oven and refrigerate for at least 4 hours or until fully chilled and set. Enjoy!

KETO MACAROONS

What You Need

- 1 1/2 cups shredded unsweetened coconut
- 1/2 cup almond flour
- 1/2 cup erythritol or your preferred keto-friendly sweetener
- 2 large egg whites
- 1/2 tsp vanilla extract
- Pinch of salt

How To Cook

- Preheat your oven to 325°F (160°C) and line a baking sheet with parchment paper.
- In a large mixing bowl, combine shredded coconut, almond flour, erythritol or sweetener, egg whites, vanilla extract, and a pinch of salt. Stir well to combine.
- Drop spoonfuls of the mixture onto the prepared baking sheet, forming small mounds.
- Bake in the preheated oven for 15-18 minutes, or until the macaroons are lightly golden on the edges.
- Remove from the oven and let the macaroons cool on the baking sheet for a few minutes.
- Transfer the macaroons to a wire rack to cool completely.
- Once cooled, store in an airtight container in the refrigerator for best freshness.
- These Keto Macaroons are a delicious and easy-to-make treat that's perfect for satisfying your sweet tooth on a keto diet.

KETO MINT CHIP BREAKFAST SMOOTHIE

What You Need

- 1/2 avocado
- 1/2 cup unsweetened coconut milk or almond milk
- 1/2 cup spinach or kale
- 1/4 cup fresh mint leaves
- 1 scoop vanilla or chocolate flavored protein powder (check for low-carb options)
- 1 tbsp unsweetened cocoa powder
- 1 tbsp powdered erythritol or stevia (or any other sugar substitute to taste)
- 1/4 tsp peppermint extract
- 1/4 tsp vanilla extract
- 1/2 cup ice cubes
- Optional: 1 tbsp cacao nibs or dark chocolate chips for "chips" in the mint chip smoothie

How To Cook

- Add all the ingredients, except for the cacao nibs or dark chocolate chips, to a blender.
- Blend on high speed until smooth and creamy.
- Taste and adjust the sweetness and mint flavor as desired.
- If desired, add the cacao nibs or dark chocolate chips to the smoothie and pulse a few times to incorporate them into the smoothie, creating a "mint chip" texture.
- Pour the smoothie into a glass and enjoy your refreshing and nutritious Keto Mint Chip Breakfast Smoothie!

KETO PUMPKIN PIE

What You Need

For the crust:

- 1 1/2 cups almond flour
- 1/4 cup coconut flour
- 1/4 cup melted butter
- 1 tbsp erythritol
- 1/2 tsp vanilla extract
- Pinch of salt

For the filling:

For the filling:

1 cup canned pumpkin puree

1/2 cup heavy cream

1/2 cup unsweetened almond milk

2 large eggs

1/2 cup erythritol

1 tsp pumpkin pie spice

1/2 tsp vanilla extract

How To Cook

- Preheat your oven to 350°F (175°C).
- In a medium bowl, combine almond flour, coconut flour, melted butter, erythritol or sweetener, vanilla extract, and a pinch of salt. Stir well until the mixture comes together.
- Press the mixture into the bottom of a greased 9-inch pie pan, evenly covering the bottom and sides to form a crust.
- Bake the crust in the preheated oven for 8-10 minutes or until lightly golden. Remove from the oven and set aside.

For the filling:

- In a large mixing bowl, whisk together the pumpkin puree, heavy cream, almond milk, eggs, erythritol or sweetener, pumpkin pie spice, vanilla extract, and a pinch of salt until well combined.
- Pour the filling mixture into the baked pie crust.
- Bake in the preheated oven for 35-40 minutes or until the center is set and a toothpick inserted in the center comes out clean.
- Remove the pie from the oven and let it cool to room temperature.
- Once cooled, refrigerate the pie for at least 2 hours before serving to allow it to set.
- Optional: Serve with whipped cream or a dollop of keto-friendly vanilla ice cream, and sprinkle with additional pumpkin pie spice for garnish.

7-11

- Hard Boiled Eggs 0g
- Beef & Cheese Sticks 1g
- 1/3 lb Big Bite Hot Dogs (No Bun) 1g
- 1/8 lb Big Bite Hot Dogs (No Bun) 1g
- Cheeseburger Bite (No Bun) 1g
- Spicy Wing Zings 3g
- Redipak Chicken Caesar Salad 5g

99 Restaurant and Pub

- Broccoli Florets 1g
- Asparagus Side 1g
- Louisiana Sirloin 2g
- Broiled Sirloin Tips 5g
- Fit For You Mushroom Bleu Top Sirloin 5g
- Fit For You Herb Salmon and Vegetables 6g
- Mushroom Bleu Top Sirloin 7g
- Fit For You Lemon Rosemary Chicken 9g

A&W Restaurants

- Broccoli Florets 1g
- Asparagus Side 1g
- Louisiana Sirloin 2g
- Broiled Sirloin Tips 5g
- Fit For You Mushroom Bleu Top Sirloin 5g
- Fit For You Herb Salmon and Vegetables 6g
- Mushroom Bleu Top Sirloin 7g
- Fit For You Lemon Rosemary Chicken 9g

Applebees

- Grilled Shrimp Skewer Salad 0g
- House Sirloin (9 Oz) 0g
- New York Strip (12 Oz) 0g
- Wings Blue Cheese Dipping Sauce 1g
- Trios Buffalo Chicken Wings - Hot 3g
- Shrimp 'N Parmesan (Topper) 4g
- Grilled Steak Caesar Salad Without Dressing (Half) 8g
- Grilled Shrimp 'N Spinach Salad Without Dressing (Regular) 13g
- Trios Buffalo Chicken Wings - Sweet & Spicy Sauce 15g
- Pecan Crusted Chicken Salad 20g

Arby's

- Cheddar Cheese Sauce (Side) 4g
- Santa Fe Ranch Dressing 4g
- Arby's Pecan Chicken Salad 5g
- Roast Turkey & Swiss Wrap (no wrap) 7g
- Roast Turkey & Swiss Sandwich (no bun) 7g
- Chopped Turkey Club Salad 7g
- Classic Roast Beef (no bun) 8g
- Double Roast Beef (no bun) 8g
- Half Pound Roast Beef (no bun) 8g
- Farmhouse Chopped Chicken Salad 8g
- Santa Fe Salad With Grilled Chicken 15g

Au Bon Pain

- Chicken Pesto Salad 0g
- Sausage Patty 0g
- Hearty Cabbage Soup Low Fat (Regular) 5g
- Hummus And Cucumber 7g
- Smoked Turkey Cobb Salad 11g
- Italian Wedding Soup (Medium) 14g
- Scrambled Eggs & Ham Breakfast Bowl 15g
- Portuguese Kale Soup (Large) 16g
- Thai Coconut Curry Soup (Medium) 18g

- Southwest Tortilla Soup (Gluten Free) (Medium) 19

Auntie Anne's

- Cheese Pretzel (No Pretzel) 1g
- DogLight Cream Cheese 1g
- Cheese Sauce 4g
- Hot Salsa Cheese 4g
- Sweet Dip 10g

Bahama Breeze

- Creole Baked Goat Cheese 0g
- Grilled Salmon 0g
- Tilapia 0g
- Jamaican Grilled Chicken Breast (Light) 1g
- Jamaican Grilled Chicken Wings 2g
- Jamaican Grilled Chicken Breast 2g
- Tomato Salsa 4g
- Broccoli 4g
- Grilled Chicken Cobb Salad 4g
- Green Beans 5g
- Vine-Ripened Tomato Salad 12g
- Breeze Salad 12g

Bar Louie

- Backyard BBQ Burger (No Bun,No BBQ) 2g
- House Salad with Dressing 10g
- Bruschetta 8g

Baskin-Robbins

- Sugar Cone 9g
- No Sugar Added Caramel Turtle Truffle 1g
- Best Sweet Cookies 'n Cream Hard Candy 12g
- Pralines 'n Cream Smooth & Creamy Hard Candy 15g

- Oreo Cookies 'N Cream Ice Cream 17g
- Old Fashioned Butter Pecan 17g
- Very Berry Strawberry Ice Cream 17g
- Cotton Candy Ice Cream 18g

Beef 'O' Brady's Pub

- Grilled Chicken Breast 0g
- Grilled Shrimp 0g
- Steak Fajitas 6g
- Grilled Shrimp Salad 9g
- Fried Mozzarella 10g
- Grilled Chicken Salad 11g
- Coleslaw 11g
- Garden Salad 13g

Benihana

- Shrimp Appetizer 0g
- Filet Mignon 1g
- Hibachi Chicken 1g
- Hibachi Steak 2g
- Japanese Onion Soup 3g
- Benihana Salad 3g
- Hibachi Shrimp 3g
- Hibachi Scallops 4g

Big Boy

- Turkey BLT Salad 5g
- Cobb Salad 8g
- Vegetable Soup 10g
- Super Big Boy (No Bread) 10g
- Chili 11g

BJ's Restaurant

- Beef Loin Strip Steak 0g
- Sirloin & Beef Patties 0g
- Boneless Skinless Chicken Breast 0g
- Smoked Salmon with 0g
- Tilapia Filets with 0g
- Reduced Sodium Bacon with 0g
- Ahi Tuna Steaks with 0g
- Pork Loin 0g
- Sirloin & Beef Patties 0g
- Broccoli Florets with 2g

Black Angus Steakhouse

- Black Angus Steakhouse Garden Salad Without Dressing
- Black Angus Steakhouse Mushroom & Bleu Filet Mignon (6 Oz)
- Black Angus Steakhouse Flame Grilled Top Sirloin (8 Oz)
- Black Angus Steakhouse Filet Mignon Center Cut (6 Oz)
- Black Angus Steakhouse Green Beans With Bacon
- Black Angus Steakhouse Grilled Asparagus
- Black Angus Steakhouse Steamed Broccoli With Parmesan Cheese
- Steak Tartare (Raw Ground Beef And Egg)

Black Bear Diner

- Bleu Cheese Dressing 2g
- Italian Green Beans 2g
- Dinner Salad 3g
- Mixed Vegetables 4g
- Shasta Scramble 8g
- Bacon Cheeseburger Salad 15g

Blaze Fast-Fire'd Pizza

- Grilled chicken 0g
- Italian sausage 0g
- Pepperoni 0g

- Salame 0g
- Smoked ham 0g
- Spicy vegan chorizo 0g
- Italian meatballs 1g
- Keto Crust 1g
- Red Vine Pizza 13g
- White Top Pizza 13g
- Veg Out 14g
- BBQ Chkn 14g
- Green Stripe Pizza 14g
- Meat Eater 14g
- Art Lover 14g
- Hot Link 15g

Bob Evans Restaurants

- Pork Sausage Links 0g
- Fully Cooked Original Pork Sausage Patties 0g
- 100% Liquid Egg Whites 0g
- Monterey Jack Cheese 0g
- Sausage Link 0g
- Sirloin Steak 3g
- Maple Pork Sausage 3g
- Cobb Salad 7g
- Border Scramble Omelet With Bob Evans Egg Lites 11g
- Farmer's Market Omelet 12g
- Garden Harvest Omelet 12g
- Wildfire Grilled Chicken Breast 14g
- Wildfire Salmon 14g

Bojangles' Famous Chicken

- Egg 0g
- Green Beans 4g
- Buffalo Bites 5g
- Fat Free Italian Dressing 5g

- Grilled Chicken Salad 6g
- Bo's Special Sauce 6g
- Chicken Breast 7g
- Roasted Chicken Bites 8g
- Chicken Leg 8g
- Chicken Thigh 8g
- Cajun Spiced Chicken Breast 12g

Bonefish Grill

- Tilapia 0g
- Rainbow Trout 0g
- Ahi Tuna Steak 0g
- French Green Beans 1g
- Chilean Sea Bass 2g
- Steamed Asparagus 2g
- Bonefish Grill Pecan Parmesan Crusted Rainbow Trout 3g
- Georges Bank Scallops & Shrimp 4g
- Fresh Greens 5g
- Lily's Chicken 6g
- Gulf Grouper Piccata 1g
- Salmon And Asparagus Salad 12g
- Sirloin & Crab Cake Dinner 12g
- Imperial Longfin 13g

Boston Market

- Award Winning Roasted Sirloin 0g
- Roasted Turkey 0g
- Beef Brisket 0g
- 3 Piece Dark Individual Meal 1g
- 1 Thigh & 1 Drumstick Individual Meal 1g
- 1/4 White Rotisserie Chicken (no Skin) 1g
- Broccoli With Garlic Butter 3g
- Green Beans (3.2 Oz) 4g
- Caesar Side Salad 5g

- Creamed Spinach 8g
- Chicken Noodle Soup 16g
- Southwest Santa Fe Salad (Half) 18g

Braum's Ice Cream

- Pork Sausage 0g
- Bacon 0g
- Half & Half 1g
- Whipped Light Cream 1g
- Mexican Style Shredded Cheese 1g
- Ultra-Pasteurized Whipping Cream 1g
- Cream Cheese 1g
- Sour Cream 2g
- Jalapeno Dip 2g
- CarbWatch Vanilla Ice Cream 3g
- 1/3 Lb Cheeseburger (No Bun) 3g
- CarbWatch Bread 7g
- Cottage Cheese 8g
- Chocolate Almond Premium Ice Cream 15g
- Fat Free No Sugar Added Strawberry Yogurt 15g

BRIO Italian Mediterranean

- New York Strip (No Mashed)
- Center Cut Filet Mignon (No Potatoes) 0g
- Grilled Salmon Fresca (No Potatoes) 4g
- Caesar 4g
- Gorgonzola Crusted Beef Medallions (No Mashed) 4g
- Lobster Bisque 10g

Buca di Beppo

- Mozzarella Caprese 2g

- Mixed Green Salad 3g
- Chicken Cacciatore 4g
- Caesar Salad 5g
- Chopped Antipasto Salad 6g
- Chicken Limone 6g
- Chicken Marsala 7g
- Mozzarella Garlic Bread 7g
- Veal Parmesan 8g
- Prosciutto Stuffed Chicken 10g
- Chicken Saltimbocca 10g
- Apple Gorgonzola Salad 13g

Buffalo Wild Wings

- Chicken Wings (1) 0g
- Sauce Spun Wings 0g
- Salt & Vinegar Traditional Wings 0g
- Knockout Punch 0g
- Grilled Chicken Breast 0g
- Jalapeno Pepper Bites 0g
- Naked Tenders (4) 0g
- Naked Tenders (6) 0g
- Traditional Wings 0g
- Grilled Chicken Club Sandwich (No Bun)
- Bacon Cheddar Burger (No Ketchup) (No Bun) 6g
- Traditional Wings-Large-Spicy Garlic 7g
- Grilled Chicken Salad 14g
- Grilled Blackened Chicken Salad 16g

Burger King

- Angus Steak Burger Patty 1g
- Whopper Patty 1g
- Hamburger Patty 1g
- Double Cheeseburger (No Bun) 1g
- Bacon Double Cheeseburger (No Bun) 1g

- Chicken Tenders (6 Pieces) 14g
- BK Chicken Fries (6 Pieces) 15g

Cafe Rio Mexican Grill

- Fire Grilled Steak 0g
- Cotija Cheese 0g
- Shredded Chicken Breast 0g
- Guacamole 0g
- Pico De Gallo 0g
- Lettuce 0g
- Fire Grilled Chicken 1g
- Cheddar Jack Blend 1g
- Chile Roasted Beef 1g
- Chicken Tostada 19g
- Fire Grilled Steak Taco 22g

California Pizza Kitchen

- Grilled Chicken Breast 0g
- Kitchen The Wedge Salad 4g
- Classic Caesar Salad With Sautéed Salmon (Half) 1g
- CPK Cobb Salad 12g
- Original Chopped Salad (Full) 12g
- Kitchen Singapore Shrimp Rolls 13g
- Lettuce Wraps Combo 14g
- Asparagus Soup Side (Cup) 14g
- Grilled Vegetable Salad 16g
- Pan-Sauteed Salmon Blackened With Wok-Stirred Vegetables 18g

Captain D's Seafood

- Grilled White Fish Fillet 0g
- Seasoned Tilapia 1g
- Broccoli 1g
- Shrimp Skewer 1g

- Side Salad 2g
- Green Beans 3g
- Scampi Butter Sauce 5g
- Stuffed Crab Shell 9g
- Chicken Tender 11g
- Wild Alaskan Salmon Salad 12g
- Country Style Fish Dinner 13g
- Cheesesticks (4 Pieces) 16g
- 3 Piece Premium Shrimp 18g

Caribou Coffee

- Cold Press Iced Coffee (Medium) 0g
- Turkey Sausage Mini (No Biscuit) 2g
- Iced Northern Lite Latte (Small) 6g
- Spinach & Mushroom Soufflé 9g
- Hot Crafted Press (Medium) 9g
- Cappuccino (Medium) 10g
- Soy Latte (Small) 11g
- Gluten Free Bacon & Gouda Soufflé 11g
- Breve (Small) 12g
- Skim Latte (Small) 12g

Carl's Jr.

- Blue Cheese Dressing 1g
- Glazed Walnuts 2g
- Buttermilk Ranch Dipping Sauce 2g
- Sausage Patty 2g
- Low Carb Breakfast Bowl 3g
- House Dressing 3g
- Chipotle Caesar Dressing 4g
- Low Fat Balsamic Dressing 5g
- Low Carb Six Dollar Burger 6g
- Low Carb Guacamole Bacon Six Dollar Burger 6g
- The Big Carl (No Bun) 7g

- Low Carb Charbroiled BBQ Chicken Sandwich 1g
- Low Carb Teriyaki Turkey Burger 15g

Carraba's Italian Grill

- Grilled Chicken (Regular) 1g
- Filet Fiorentina 1g
- Tuscan-Grilled Filet 1g
- Tuscan Grilled Chicken 1g
- Tuscan Grilled Pork Chop 1g
- Sirloin Marsala (Small) 2g
- Chicken Marsala (Small) 2g
- Chicken Marsala (Regular) 2g
- The Johnny 5g
- Sauteed Spinach 8g
- Crab Cakes 8g
- Broccoli Alla Gratinatta 9g
- Spicy Sausage & Lentil Soup 1g

Casey's General Store

- Bacon Cheeseburger (No Bun) 2g
- Southwest Roast Beef Wrap 3g
- Raw Almonds 3g
- Hot & Spicy Peanuts 3g
- Teriyaki Beef Jerky 6g
- Chef Salad 9g
- Ham & Egg Croissant 18g
- Chicken Tenders (3) 24g

Charleys Philly Steaks

- Grilled Chicken Salad 8g
- Chicken Teriyaki Salad 10g

- Buffalo Chicken Salad 1g
- Chicken Fingers (5) 15g

Checkers

- Extra Hot Classic Wings (5 Piece) 1g
- Parmesan Garlic Classic Wings (5 Piece) 1g
- Baconzilla (No Bun) 2g
- Rallyburger With Cheese (No Bun) 2g
- Medium Buffalo Classic Wings (5 Piece) 2g
- Parmesan Garlic Classic Wings (10 Piece) 2g

Cheddar's Scratch Kitchen

- Chicken Tenders 0g
- Salmon 0g
- Broccoli 2g
- Ribeye 6g
- Sweet Baby Carrots 8g
- Grilled Chicken Pecan Salad 8g
- Lemon Pepper Chicken 9g
- House Salad without Dressing 9g
- Broccoli Cheese Casserole 14g

Chick-Fil-A

- 8-count Grilled Chicken Nuggets 1g
- Grilled Chicken Sandwich (without bun): 3g
- Grilled Chicken Club Sandwich (without bun): 3g
- Grilled Nuggets (eight count): 3g
- Bacon Egg & Cheese Biscuit (ask for no biscuit) 3g
- Grilled Cobb Salad (ask for no corn) 15g

Chili's Grill & Bar

- Flame-Grilled Ribeye 1g
- Grilled Chicken Platter 2g
- Spicy Garlic & Lime Grilled Shrimp Combo 4g
- Wings Over Buffalo With Bleu Cheese Dressing 5g
- Guacamole, Sour Cream, Cheese & Pico De Gallo (Boat) 5g
- Caesar Salad (Side) 1g
- Classic Chicken Fajitas 12g

Chipotle Mexican Grill

- Guacamole (4 Oz) 2g
- Sour Cream 2g
- Fajita Vegetables 4g
- Cauliflower Rice 4g
- Keto Salad Bowl - Steak 7g
- Keto Bowl 7g
- Paleo Bowl 1g
- Whole30 Bowl 12g

Chuck E Cheese

- 100% Natural String Cheese 1g
- Buffalo Wings 3g
- Celery & Bleu Cheese 4g
- Veggie Platter 5g
- Side Fruit Garnish 8g
- Carrot Sticks with Ranch 10g
- Cinnamon Sticks 1g
- 24 Piece Wing Platter 12g
- Mandarin Oranges 14g

Church's Chicken

- Original Breast 2g
- Original Leg 3g
- Spicy Tender Strips 3g
- Original Wing 4g
- Original Thigh 4g
- Tender Strips 6g
- Spicy Leg 7g
- Spicy Breast 10g
- Nuggets 12g
- Premium Homestyle Fillet 14g

Chuy's

- Crispy Beef Taco 6g
- Chile Rellenos 7g
- Creamy Jalapeno Sauce 8g
- Grilled Chicken Salad 12g
- Beef Enchilada 12g
- Mexican Rice with 20g of net carbs
- Mexi-Cobb Salad with 20g of net carbs

Cicis

- Chicken Noodle Soup 6g
- 12" Ole Buffet Pizza 10g
- Chicken Bacon Club 13g
- 12" Zesty Veggie Buffet Pizza 15g
- 12" Zesty Ham & Cheddar Buffet Pizza 16g
- 12" Zesty Tomato Alfredo Buffet Pizza 16g
- Thin Crust Italiano 16g
- 12" Bacon Cheddar Buffet Pizza 16g

Cinnabon

- Cinnamon Almonds 12g
- Cinnamon Mixed Nuts 12g

- Jalapeño Cheddar Sausage Bites 15g
- Cinnamon Cashews 15g
- Cinnamon Bread 19g
- Cinnamon Bread with Cinnamon Bursts 19g
- Mini Pull-Aparts 19g
- Cinnamon Sandwich Cookies 19g

Circle K

- Cheeseburger Dog (No Bun) 1g
- Beef Jerky 1g
- Sea Salt Roasted Almonds 4g
- Garden Salad 5g

Cold Stone Creamery

- Chocolate Chips Mix-In 2g
- Raspberries 4g
- Peanut Butter Mix-In 4g
- Rainbow Sprinkles 6g
- Chocolate Shavings 7g
- Strawberries 7g
- Smooth Cravings 70 Calorie Hot Cocoa Mix 8g
- Yellow Cake 13g

Cooper's Hawk Restaurant

- Grilled Medallions 0g
- Asparagus 3g
- Blackened Bleu Skirt Steak 4g
- Seared Salmon 6g
- BBQ Ranch Chicken Salad (No BBQ) 6g

Corner Bakery Cafe

- Pickle Spear 1g
- Tuna Salad (Trio Size) 2g

- Egg Salad (Trio Size) 3g
- Anaheim Scrambler with Egg Whites 4g
- Farmer's Scrambler with Egg Whites 5g
- Caesar Salad (Trio) 6g
- Asian Edamame Salad (Trio Size) 6g
- Anaheim Scrambler 6g

Costco

- Frozen Chicken Breast 0g
- New York Strip Steak 0g
- Langostino Lobster Tails 0g
- Rotisserie Chicken 0g
- Rotisserie Chicken Salad 0g
- Salmon Milano With Basil Pesto Butter 1g
- Pork Tenderloin 1g
- Hot Italian Sausage 1g
- Hot Dog (No Bun) 5g
- Pork Belly Sous Vide 5g
- Chicken Caesar Salad 6g
- Turkey & Swiss Roller 8g
- Chicken Salad Sonoma 13g
- Toasted Coconut Cashews 16g

Cracker Barrel

- Sharp White Cheddar 0g
- Sharp Cheddar Cheese 0g
- Extra Sharp Cheddar Cheese Sticks 0g
- Extra Sharp Cheddar Cheese Cracker Cuts 0g
- Extra Sharp White Cheddar Cheese 0g
- Jalapeño Cheddar 0g
- Extra Sharp Cheddar Cheese Cuts 0g
- Sharp Cheddar Cheese Sticks 0g
- Campfire Chicken Lunch Meat 1g
- Pan Roasted Turkey Breast Deli Meat 1g

- Roast Beef 10g

Culver's

- Unsweetened Iced Tea 0g
- Ground Beef Patty (Single) 0g
- Tea (Hot) 0g
- Dill Pickles (Sliced) 0g
- Bacon (Slice) 0g
- Chicken Cashew With Grilled Chicken Salad 1g
- Caesar With Flame Roasted Chicken Salad 1g
- Chicken Noodle Soup 13g
- Chicken Cashew With Flame Roasted Chicken Salad 13g

Dairy Queen

- Sausage (2 Patties) 0g
- Bacon (3 Slices) 1g
- Almond Pieces 1g
- Side Salad 3g
- Hot Dog No Ketchup (No Bun) 3g
- Cheeseburger (No Bun) 4g
- Double Cheeseburger (No Bun) 4g
- Coconut Flakes 5g
- Grilled Chicken Salad 7g
- Grilled Chicken BLT Salad 7g
- Chicken Fingers (2 Fingers) 13g

Dave & Buster's

- 14 oz Ribeye 0g
- Grilled Steak Salad
- Crispy cauliflower

Del Frisco's Double Eagle

- USDA Prime Chopped Steak 2g

- Jumbo Shrimp Cocktail 2g
- Roasted wings 2g
- Tuna Tartare 2g
- Pan Roasted Salmon 2g
- Chilled Lobster Cocktail 2g
- Sticky Garlic Ribs 8g
- Del's Jumbo Lump Crab Cake 12g
- The Grille Salad 12g

Del Taco

- Side Of Bacon 0g
- Bacon Double Del Cheeseburger 4g
- Taco 8g
- Taco Salad 8g
- Mini Bacon Quesadilla 13g
- Grilled Chicken Taco 14g
- Steak Taco Del Carbon 17g
- Chicken Bacon Avocado Salad 18g

Denny's

- Grilled Shrimp Skewer (1) 0g
- Eggs 1g
- Grilled Ham Slice 1g
- Senior Grilled Chicken Breast 2g
- T-bone Steak & Eggs 4g
- Cottage Cheese 5g
- Ultimate Omelette 6g
- Fit-Fare Grilled Chicken Breast Salad With Lemon Or Lime Wedges 1g
- Prime Rib Skillet 12g

Dickey's Barbecue Pit

- Turkey Breast 0g
- Turkey 0g

- Ham 0g
- Olive Vinaigrette Dressing 0g
- Fried Onion Tanglers 0g
- Breakfast Ham 1g
- Hot Links 1g
- Low Carb Barbecue Sauce 1g
- Pulled Pork 2g
- Caesar Salad Without Croutons 2g
- Half Chicken 2g
- Chicken 8g

Domino's

- Ranch Dipping Sauce 2g
- Hot Buffalo Wings 3g
- Buffalo Chicken Kickers 3g
- Boneless Chicken 3g
- Sweet Mango Habanero Chicken Wings 3g
- BBQ Chicken Wings 3g
- Plain Wings 3g
- Hot Wings 3g
- Regular Specialty Chicken - Sweet BBQ Bacon 5g
- Regular Specialty Chicken - Classic Hot Buffalo 5g
- Pizza Breadsticks 1 Stick 1g
- Mighty Meaty Pizza 1 Slice 18g

Donatos Pizza

- Italian Garden Side Salad 3g
- Tuscan Chicken Caesar Salad 3g
- Side Harvest Salad 1g
- Chicken Spinach Mozzarella No Dough Pizza 14g
- Pepperoni No Dough Pizza 15g

Dunkin' Donuts

- Egg & Cheese (No Bun) 1g
- Bacon, Egg White & Cheese (No Bun) 1g
- DD Smart Egg & Cheese (No Bun) 1g
- Ham, Egg & Cheese (No Bun) 1g
- Sausage Egg & Cheese (No Bun) 1g
- DD Smart Egg White & Cheese (No Bun) 1g
- Bacon, Egg & Cheese (No Bun) 1g
- Ham, Egg White & Cheese (No Bun) 1g
- Sausage, Egg White & Cheese (No Bun) 1g
- Egg White Veggie (No Bun) 1g
- Egg White Turkey Sausage (No Bun) 1g
- Turkey Sausage (No Bun) 1g
- Iced Coffee With Cream (Small) 3g
- Lite Garden Vegetable Cream Cheese 5g

Einstein Bros. Bagels

- Caesar Dressing 1g
- Turkey Sausage 1g
- Whipped Plain Cream Cheese 1g
- Hummus 2g
- Whipped Plain Reduced Fat Cream Cheese 2g
- Spicy Roasted Tomato Spread 2g
- Roasted Tomato Spread 2g
- Whipped Smoked Salmon Cream Cheese 2g
- Candied Walnuts 6g
- Creamy Peanut Butter 8g
- Chicken Noodle Soup 13g
- Chicken Caesar Salad 13g
- Broccoli Sharp Cheddar (Cup) 14g
- Chicken Club Salad 17g
- Bagels Chipotle Chicken Salad 18g
- Asiago Chicken Caesar Salad 18g

El Pollo Loco

- Flame Grilled Chicken Breast, Skinless 0g
- Flame Grilled Chicken Breast 0g
- Flame Grilled Chicken Leg 0g
- Flame Grilled Chicken Thigh 0g
- Flame Grilled Chicken Wing 0g
- Flame Grilled Chicken Chopped Breast Meat
- Loco Garden Salad 1g
- Broccoli 4g
- Skinless Chicken Breast Meal 8g
- The World's First Keto Burrito 10g
- Avocado Salad 14g
- Grilled Chicken Salad (No Dressing) 15g
- Double Chicken Power Bowl 15g

Famous Dave's

- Pineapple Rage Hot Sauce 2g
- Buffalo Chicken Wings 2g
- Wilburs Revenge 2g
- Collard Greens 2g
- Signature Spicy Pickle Relish 4g
- St. Louis Ribs 4g
- Firecracker Green Beans 4g
- Hot Link Sausage 4g

Fazoli's

- Caesar Dressing 1g
- Broccoli 2g
- Caesar Side Salad 2g
- Broccoli 2g
- Ranch Dressing 2g
- Creamy Parmesan Peppercorn Ranch 2g
- Grilled Chicken 2g
- Sliced Italian Sausage 3g
- Red Wine Vinaigrette 3g

- Broccoli and Fire Roasted Tomatoes 3g
- Italian Side Salad 3g
- Garden Side Salad 4g
- Meatballs 5g
- Chicken Artichoke Salad 7g
- Antipasto Salad 8g

Firebirds Wood Fired Grill

- 7 Oz Filet 0g
- Smoked Chicken Wings 0g
- Broccoli 2g
- Wood Grilled Salmon 5g
- Spiced Pecan Green Beans 6g
- BLT Salad (Small) 7g
- Sauteed Spinach 7g
- Ahi Tuna Appetizer 7g
- Mixed Vegetables 8g
- Cilantro Chicken 14g

Firehouse Subs

- Firehouse Chopped Salad (No Meat) 6g
- Italian Chopped Salad With Grilled Chicken 11g
- Chopped Salad With Grilled Chicken 12g
- Chief's Salad With Chicken 12g
- Chief's Salad With Turkey 14g
- Chicken Noodle Soup (Small) 16g

First Watch

- Mushroom & Cheese Omelet 3g
- Far West Omelet 4g
- Denver Melt with 4g of net carbs
- Ham & Gruyere Omelet with 4g
- Bacado Omelet 5g

- Pecan Dijon Salad 6g
- Greek Fetish Omelet 6g
- Cobb Salad 7g
- Lean Machine 7g
- Joaquin Yahoo 7g
- Acapulco Express Omelet 15g

Five Guys Burgers and Fries

- Patrick Cudahy Bacon 0g
- Bunless Bacon Burger 1g
- Bunless Cheeseburger 1g
- Bunless Bacon Cheese Dog 1g
- Bunless Little Cheeseburger 1g
- Bunless Little Bacon Burger 1g
- Mt. Olive Fresh Kosher Dill Pickles 1g

Flemings

- Chilled Seafood Tower (without ahi tuna poke and lavash crackers)
- Beef Carpaccio (without crostini)
- Burrata with Prosciutto (without croutons)
- Shrimp Cocktail
- Seared Pork Belly (without fig demi-glace)
- Petite Filet Mignon 8oz
- Main Filet Mignon 11oz
- Certified Angus Beef Ribeye 14oz
- Prime Bone-In Ribeye 20oz
- Prime New York Strip 16oz
- Prime Tomahawk 35oz
- Prime Dry Aged Ribeye 16oz
- Roasted Asparagus
- Cauliflower Mash
- Roasted Asparagus

Fogo de Chao

- PICANHA
- FILET MIGNON
- BEEF ANCHO
- COSTELA DE PORCO
- FRANGO
- LINGUIÇA
- CHILLED LOBSTER AND SHRIMP APPETIZER
- COLD WATER LOBSTER APPETIZER
- SMOKED SALMON

Freddy's Frozen Custard

- Grilled Chicken Breast (Lettuce Wrapped) 3g
- Steakburger with Cheese (Lettuce Wrapped) 3g
- California Steakburger (Lettuce Wrapped) 8g
- Hot Dog (Lettuce Wrapped) 1g
- Chili Cheese Dog (Lettuce Wrapped) 12g

Friendly's

- Bacon 0g
- Hot Dog (No Bun) 2g
- Broccoli (Side) 2g
- Grilled Chicken Breast 2g
- Side Salad 8g
- No Sugar Added Vanilla Ice Cream 8g
- Mixed Vegetables (Side) 9g
- Clam Chowder 1g
- 2+2 Grilled Flounder 13g
- Premium Purely Pistachio Ice Cream 1/2 cup 16g
- Chicken Strips (Kid's) 17g
- 2+2 Kickin Buffalo Chicken Strips 20g

Fuddruckers

- Elk Patty 0g

- 1/3 lb Beef Patty 0g
- Turkey Patty 0g
- Grilled Chicken Breast 0g
- Swiss Cheese 1g
- Pepper Jack Cheese 1g
- Southwest Burger 6g
- Cheese Sauce 6g
- Market Toss Salad 6g

Fuzzy's Taco Shop

- Shredded Beef Soft Taco 12g
- Shredded Chicken Soft Taco 12g
- Grilled Fish Taco 13g
- Avocado Ranch Dressing 13g
- Grilled Shrimp Taco 14g
- Big Salad Shredded Chicken 19g
- Grilled Shrimp Salad 19g
- Shredded Brisket Salad 20g

Godfather's Pizza

- Wings 0g
- Cheese Thin Crust Pizza (1 Slice) 14g
- Pepperoni Thin Crust Pizza (1 Slice) 14g
- Taco Thin Crust Pizza (1 Slice) 15g
- Humble Pie Thin Crust Pizza (1 Slice) 15g
- Hawaiian Thin Crust Pizza (1 Slice) 15g
- Veggie Thin Crust Pizza (1 Slice) 15g

Golden Chick

- Golden Roast Chicken Thigh 0g
- Roasted Wing 1g
- Golden Roast Leg 1g
- Golden Roast Chicken Breast 1g

- Village Ranch Dressing 1g
- Wing 2g
- Side Salad 3g
- Green Beans 5g
- Chicken Tenders 15g
- Fried Catfish 6g
- Golden Chick'N Nuggets 15g
- Chicken Salad Salad 18g

Golden Corral

- Rotisserie Chicken (Breast & Wing) 0g
- Whole Carved Salmon 0g
- Bacon 0g
- Baked New Orleans Style Fish 0g
- Sausage Patty 0g
- Rotisserie Chicken (Breast & Wing) 0g
- Rotisserie Chicken 0g
- Romaine Lettuce 1g
- Baked Florentine Fish 1g
- Sirloin Steak 1g
- Green Beans 2g
- Maryland-Style Crab Cakes 7g
- Seafood Salad (1/2 Cup) 7g

Hard Rock Cafe

- Grilled chicken topped with bacon with Monterey jack cheese melted over it, with fajita vegetables as a side order
- Grilled chicken (Hold the marinade and seasoning)
- Grilled salmon (Hold the marinade and seasoning)
- Steak burger patty
- Grilled shrimp (Hold the marinade and seasoning)
- Fajita grilled steak, chicken, shrimp (Hold the marinade and seasoning)
- Bacon
- Avocado

Hardee's

- Sausage Patty 1g
- Low Carb Breakfast Bowl 2g
- 2/3 lb Monster Thickburger (No Bun) 2g
- Buttermilk Ranch Dipping Sauce 3g
- Fat Free Italian Dressing 3g
- 1/3 lb Low Carb Thickburger 4g
- Low Carb Little Thickburger 5g
- Side Salad (No Dressing) 5g
- Low Carb Charbroiled Chicken Club Sandwich 13g

Hooters

- Naked Chicken Wing 0g
- Naked Chicken Wings 0g
- Sugar Free Lite Energy Drink 0g
- Medium Wing Sauce 1g
- Steamed Shrimp 1g
- Snow Crab Legs 1g
- Hot Wing Sauce 1g
- Extra Hot 3 Mile Island Wing Sauce 1g
- Raw Oysters (Dozen) 7g
- Garden Salad (Side) 10g
- Grilled Chicken Garden Salad 19g

Houlihans

- Houlihan's Heartland Grilled Chicken Salad 20 Carbs
- Houlihan's Grilled Shrimp Azteca 15 Carbs
- Houlihan's Mediterranean Orzo 20 Carbs
- Houlihan's Seared Sea Scallops 10 Carbs
- Houlihan's Grilled 4 Oz Atlantic Salmon 10 Carbs
- Houlihan's Grilled Asparagus 5 Carbs
- Houlihan's Grilled Asparagus Salad 5 Carbs

Huddle House

- Grilled Chicken 0g
- Unsweetened Tea 0g
- Hot Tea 0g
- Hometown Blend Coffee 1g
- Ribeye 6oz 2g
- Sugar Cured Ham 3g
- Ham and Cheese Omelette 6g
- Turkey Chef Salad 1g
- Philly Cheesesteak Omelette w/ American Cheese 12g
- Bacon Cheddar Grits 17g
- Stuffed and Smothered Omelette Chicken Tenders 18g

Hungry Howie's Pizza

- Howie Wings 0g
- Ranch Dressing 1g
- Italian Dressing 2g
- Antipasto Salad (Small) 2g
- Greek Salad Dressing 2g
- Chef Salad (Small) 5g
- Marinara Dipping Sauce 8g
- Chef Salad (Large) 8g
- Thin Crust Pepperoni Pizza 1 Slice 9g

IHOP

- Pork Sausage Links 1g
- Mushrooms 2g
- Green Peppers & Onions 2g
- Simple & Fit House Salad 6g
- Garden Omelette 13g
- Turkey Bacon Omelette For Me 15g
- Hearty Ham & Cheese Omelette 16g

- Simple & Fit Grilled Tilapia 19g

In-N-Out Burger

- Flying Dutchman 0g
- Meat Patty 0g
- Cheese Slice 0g
- Double-Double Protein Style (No Spread) 8g
- Cheeseburger Protein Style 8g
- Double-Double Protein Style 8g
- 4X4 Protein Style 8g

Jack in the Box

- Fried Egg 0g
- Breakfast Jack (No Bun) 1g
- Ultimate Cheeseburger (No Bun Or Ketchup) 2g
- Box Bacon Ultimate Cheeseburger (No Bun) 2g
- Fresh Brewed Iced Tea (20 Fl Oz) 2g
- Side Salad 2g
- Sourdough Grilled Chicken Club (No Bun) 4g
- Hearty Breakfast Bowl (No Hash Browns) 5g
- Grilled Chicken Strips 5g
- Acapulco Chicken Salad With Grilled Chicken Strips 10g
- Spicy Chicken Sandwich (No Bun) 15g
- Asian Chicken Salad With Grilled Chicken Strips 16g
- Chicken Breast Strips (2) 16g
- Cheesy Macaroni Bites (3 Pieces) 19g
- Mozzarella Cheese Sticks (3) 20g
- Southwest Grilled Chicken Salad 21g

Jack's

- Green Beans 5g
- Grits 6g
- Double Cheese Burger (No Bun) 6g

- Hard Cider 1g
- Grilled Chicken Salad 1g
- Chicken Fingers 12g
- Sausage, Egg & Cheese Wrap 23g

Jamba Juice

- Wheatgrass Detox Shot (2 Oz) 2g
- Ginger Shot 5g
- Razzmatazz Smoothie 12g
- Turkey, Dijon & Jack Mini Wrap 13g
- Apple 'N Greens 15g
- Frozen Fruit Sorbet Bars - Peach BlackBerry Smash 15g
- Tropical Fruit+Mania 18g
- Zesty Southwest Grilled Chicken Salad 19g

Jason's Deli

- Dill Pickle Spear 0g
- Premium Ham Slimwich (1/2 Portion) 0g
- Provolone (1 Slice) 0g
- Extra Virgin Olive Oil 0g
- Imported Finlandia Swiss (1 Slice) 0g
- Grilled Chicken Breast 0g
- Hot Corned Beef Slimwich 0g
- Hot New York Style Pastrami Slimwich 0g
- Smoked Red Pepper-Cilantro Aioli 0g
- Chicken Strips 1g
- Roasted Turkey Breast 1g
- French Onion Soup (Cup) 9g
- Big Chef Salad 1g
- Broccoli Cheese Soup (Cup) 12g
- Clam Chowder (Cup) 16g

Jersey Mike's Subs

- Chef Salad 7g
- #7 Turkey Breast & Provolone (In A Tub) 7g
- #8 Club Sub (In A Tub) 10g
- #5 Super Sub (In A Tub) 11g
- #13 Original Italian (In A Tub) 12g
- #17 Steak Philly (In A Tub) 13g
- #43 Chipotle Steak (In A Tub) 16g

Jimmy John's

- Jumbo Kosher Dill Pickle with 0g of net carbs
- Iced Tea (Large) with 0g of net carbs
- Iced Tea (Small) with 0g of net carbs
- Lettuce with 0g of net carbs
- Italian Vinaigrette with 0g of net carbs
- #10 Hunter's Club Unwich (No Mayo) 2g
- #7 Gourmet Smoked Ham Club Unwich 4g
- #12 Beach Club Unwich (No Mayo) 7g
- #9 Italian Night Club Unwich 8g

Joe's Crab Shack

- Dipping Butter 0g
- Crab Cake Chipotle Caesar 0g
- Snow Crab Legs 0g
- Spicy Boil 1g
- Broccoli Florets 3g
- Joe's Classic Steampot 4g
- Side Salad 6g
- Bucket of Shrimp (12) 7g
- Joe's Famous BBQ with 8g
- New England Clam Chowder 20g

Johnny Rockets

- Patty Melt (No Bun) 1g
- Garden Salad 5g
- Tuna Melt (No Bread) 8g
- Onion Rings 18g
- Grilled Chicken Club Salad 18g
- Rocket Single 30g
- Grilled Cheese 40g

KFC

- Grilled Chicken Whole Wing 0g
- Fiery Grilled Wings 0g
- Lipton Brisk Green with Peach Tea (16 oz) 0g
- Buttery Spread with 0g of net carbs
- Grilled Boneless Filet 0g
- Colonel's Buttery Spread 0g
- Hot Wings (1) 3g
- Original Recipe Chicken Wing 3g
- Original Recipe Chicken Whole Wing 5g
- Fried Chicken Breast & Wing (White Meat) 17g

Krispy Kreme Doughnuts

- Mini Original Glazed Doughnut 10g
- Doughnut Bites 20g
- Chocolate Doughnut Bites 21g
- Strawberry Iced Glazed Doughnut 22g
- Blueberry Mini Crullers 28g

Krystal

- 4Carb Scrmblr (Sausage) 1g
- Low Carb Scrambler 2g
- Low Carb Scrambler (Bacon) 2g
- 4Carb Scrmblr (Bacon) 3g
- Chik'n Bites Salad 8g

- Fries (Small) 12g
- Plain Pup with 14g
- Bacon Cheese Krystal 14g

La Madeleine Cafe

- Egg Crepe Champignon 0g
- Caesar Dressing 1g
- Steamed Asparagus 1g
- Spinach Salade (Petite) 2g
- Balsamic Vinaigrette 3g
- Rotisserie Half Chicken with Skin 5g
- Fat Free Caesar Dressing 5g
- Petite Caesar-Fat Free Dressing 7g
- Rotisserie Whole Chicken With Skin 9g
- Green Beans Almondine 9g
- Chicken Caesar Salad (Regular) 15g

Lazy Dog Restaurant

- Veggie Lavosh Sandwich 0g
- Caesar Dressing 3g
- Cobb Salad 7g
- Chicken Lettuce Wraps 8g
- Grilled Garlic Flatbread 13g
- Japanese Cucumber Salad 13g
- Hawaiian Pizza 15g
- Sundried Tomato Spinach Dip 16g
- Sesame Crusted Ahi Tuna 17g
- Chicken Tenders 17g

Lees

- Grilled Chicken Breast
- Green Beans
- Coleslaw

- Salad

Legal Sea Foods

- Salad Shrimp 0g
- New England Clam Chowder 9g
- Cocktail Sauce 10g
- Lobster Bisque 12g
- Crab & Sweet Corn Chowder 20g
- Shrimp Risotto 22g
- Popcorn Shrimp 27g

Little Caesars Pizza

- Oven Roasted Wings 0g
- Buttery Garlic Dip 0g
- Caesar Salad Dressing 1g
- Garlic Parmesan Wings 1g
- Mild Wings 1g
- Cheezy Jalapeno Dip 2g
- Chipotle Dip 2g
- Ranch Dip 3g
- Buffalo Wings 3g
- Antipasto Salad 6g
- Greek Salad 8g

Logan's Roadhouse

- Sirloin (10 oz) 0g
- Filet Mignon 0g
- Sirloin (6 oz) 0g
- Santa Fe Tilapia 0g
- Chopped Sirloin 0g
- Mesquite Grilled Salmon 0g
- Health Nut Grilled Chicken Salad 0g
- Parmesan Peppercorn Salad Dressing 2g

- Health Nut Side Salad 2g
- Mesquite Wood Grilled Chicken Salad 2g
- Steamed Broccoli 3g
- House Salad (No Dressing) 4g
- Sauteed Mushrooms 4g
- Health Nut Filet Mignon Meal 8g
- Grilled Vegetable Skewer 10g
- Roadhouse Salad - Sirloin 18g

Long John Silver's

- Baked Cod 1g
- Freshside Grille Shrimp Scampi 1g
- Freshside Grille Vegetable Medley (Side) 5g
- Broccoli Cheese Soup 7g
- Battered Chicken Plank 9g
- Breaded Mozzarella Sticks 12g
- Battered Fish 13g
- Lobster Stuffed Crab Cake 15g

LongHorn Steakhouse

- Cowboy Pork Chop (Lunch) with 0g
- Flat Iron Steak 0g
- Ribeye (12 oz) 0g
- Eye of Prime Rib with Au Jus (12 oz) 0g
- Eye of Prime Rib with Au Jus (16 oz) 0g
- Renegade Top Sirloin (12 oz) 0g
- Flo's Filet & Lobster Tail 0g
- Lobster Tail 0g
- Redrock Grilled Shrimp (Dinner) 2g
- Baby Back Ribs (Half-Rack)2g
- Sierra Chicken (Dinner) 2g
- Big Sky Bleu Filet (7 Oz) 5g
- Sirloin & Shrimp Scampi 6g

Luby's Cafeteria

- Roasted Chicken (Half) 0g
- Grilled Chicken Breast 0g
- Grilled Chicken Breast without Skin 1g
- Ranch Dressing 1g
- Turkey Chopped Steak 2g
- Spinach Salad 2g
- Spring Mix Salad 2g
- Bacon Cheese Steak 2g
- Angus Chopped Steak 3g
- Blackened Tilapia 3g
- Fresh Green Beans 6g
- Fried Fish 1/2 14g

Maggiano's Little Italy

- Fresh Grilled Asparagus 3g
- Maggiano's Salad 7g
- Tuscan & Sausage Orzo Soup (Cup) 8g
- Meatball 9g
- Chicken Francese 1g
- Tomato Caprese 13g
- Chicken Saltimbocca 13g
- Chopped Salad 13g

Marco's Pizza

- Chicken Dippers 4g
- Meatball Bake 5g
- Chicken Ranch Salad 7g
- All Meat Pizza Bowl 9g
- Deluxe Pizza Bowl 1g
- CinnaSquares 1g
- Cheesy Bread 1g

- Garden Pizza Bowl 1g

Mastro's Steakhouse Ocean Club

- Shrimp Cocktail 0g
- Oysters on Halfshell 0g
- A5 WAGYU BEEF ROLL 0g
- Crispy Garlic Tuna Sashimi 0g
- Tomahawk 0g
- Jumbo Lump Crab Cakes 8g
- Lobster Bisque 15g
- New England Clam Chowder 15g
- ALL STEAK AND CHICKEN
- Asparagus 2g
- Broccoli 2g

McAlister's Deli

- Pickle Spear 0g
- Butter Packet 0g
- Comeback Gravy 1g
- Blue Cheese Salad Dressing 1g
- Lite Ranch Salad Dressing 1g
- Ranch Salad Dressing 1g
- Meatloaf with Gravy 1g
- Garden Salad With Chicken Salad 9g
- Broccoli Cheddar Soup 1g
- Chicken & Sausage Gumbo 15g
- Greek Chicken Salad 16g
- Southwest Cobb Salad 20g

McDonalds

- Sausage Patty 1g
- Applewood Smoked Bacon 1g
- Canadian Bacon: 1g

- Folded Egg: 1g
- Egg: 1g
- American Cheese 1g
- Egg McMuffin w/ Canadian Bacon (No Muffin) 3g
- Sausage, Egg & Cheese McMuffin (No Muffin) 3g
- Bacon, Egg & Cheese Biscuit (No Biscuit) 4g
- Quarter Pounder w/ Cheese & Bacon (No Bun) 4g
- Big Mac (No Sauce, No Bun) 4g
- Premium Bacon Ranch Salad With Grilled Chicken 7g
- Bacon Ranch Salad With Grilled Chicken (with Ranch Dressing) 1g
- Chicken McNuggets (6 Pieces) (No Sauce) 15g

Miller's Ale House

- Wings 5g
- Chicken Philly (No Bun) 4g
- Zingers 18g
- Zinger Salad 23g
- Blackened Shrimp & Chicken Cobb Salad 33g

Mimi's Bistro & Bakery

- Mahi Mahi 0g
- Broiled Salmon 0g
- Smoked Bacon and Eggs 1g
- Espresso 1g
- Broccoli 2g
- Ranch Dressing 2g
- Egg Whites 2g
- Mini Wedge 3g
- Monterey Omelette 4g
- Five Alarm Santa Fe Egg White Omelette 4g
- French Market Onion Soup 14g
- Asian Chopped Salad 16g
- Chicken And Fruit Salad 18g
- Grilled Beef Liver 24g

MOD Pizza

- Mild Sausage 0g
- Artichokes 0g
- Mozzarella Cheese w/1g
- White Sauce 1g
- Red Sauce 1g
- Grilled Chicken 1g
- Canadian Bacon 1g
- Mod Spinach 1g
- Roasted Broccoli 2g
- Mad Dog Pizza 1 slice 1g
- Deluxe Salad 12g
- Greek Salad 18g

Moe's Southwest Grill

- Steak with 0g of net carbs
- Cheese with 0g of net carbs
- Chunky Guacamole with 1g of net carbs
- Chicken 1g
- Streaker Moo Moo Mr. Cow - Chicken 5g
- Streaker Moo Moo Mr. Cow - Steak 5g
- Streaker Alfredo Garcia Fajita - Steak 14g
- Personal Trainer Streaker - Veg 15g
- Close Talker Streaker Salad - Fish 15g
- Close Talker Streaker Salad - Chicken 16g
- Close Talker Streaker Salad - Steak 18g
- Close Talker Streaker Salad - Ground Beef 19g
- Close Talker Streaker Salad - Pork 20g

Morton's The Steakhouse

- Best Low Carb Entree at Mortons Steakhouse:

- Espresso crusted Zabuton steak with garlic cream and gremolata, sautéed brussels sprouts cooked plain with no sauce.
- Ahi tuna tower (no sauce, tuna marinade)
- Bacon wrapped sea scallops
- Maine lobster tail
- Colossal crab meat cocktail
- Jumbo shrimp cocktail
- Nueske's bacon wrapped steak (no glaze, plain)
- Angus steak, all cuts (no au jus, served plain)
- Oysters on the half shell
- Baseball cut sirloin steak, black and blue (no au jus, onion)
- Prosciutto wrapped mozzarella (no balsamic glaze or vinaigrette)
- Red king crab legs USDA prime steak, all cuts (no au jus)
- Ora king salmon (no balsamic glaze)
- Coulotte steak, porcini dusted, wild mushrooms (no au jus,
- SRF wagyu gold Manhattan (no au jus)
- Miso marinated sea bass (no miso)
- Smoked gouda cheese
- Blue cheese
- Parmesan cheese
- Sautéed brussels sprouts (no sauce, serve plain)
- Jumbo asparagus (served plain, no hollandaise sauce)
- Sautéed broccoli florets (no bread crumbs)

Mountain Mike's Pizza

- Plain Wings 0g
- Frank's RedHot Wings 0g
- Salad 4g
- Mozzarella Sticks 10g

Newk's Eatery

- Chicken Salad 0g
- Cobb Salad 2g
- Fat Free Ranch 3g

- Shrimp & Avocado Salad 7g
- Chicken Chili 8g
- Shrimp Remoulade Salad 9g
- Greek Salad 10g
- Broccoli Cheese Soup 11g
- Simply Salad 16g
- Ultimate Salad 17g

Noodles & Company

- Grilled Chicken 0g
- Grilled Chicken Breast 0g
- Seasoned Chicken 0g
- Sauteed Shrimp 0g
- Braised Beef 0g
- Braised Pork 0g
- Chicken Breast 0g
- Sauteed Beef (Small) 0g
- Marinated Steak 1g
- Tossed Green Salad 2g
- Asparagus Stack 2g
- Meatballs 3g
- Parmesan-Crusted Chicken Breast 8g
- Tomato Basil Bisque (Side) 11g
- Buff Tuscan Fresca 12g
- Backyard BBQ Chicken Salad (Small) 16g

O'Charley's

- Sausage (2 Patties) 0g
- Flame-Grilled Top Sirloin (10 oz) 0g
- Your Favorite Ribeye Steak 0g
- Bacon (1 Slice) 0g
- Jr. Grilled Chicken 0g
- Grilled Top Sirloin 0g
- O'Charley's Butchers Cut Premium USDA Choice Steak (5 oz) 0g

- Jr. Grilled Steak 0g
- Classic Caesar Salad 13g
- Cajun Chicken Salad 13g

Old Chicago Pizza and Taproom

- Antipasto Salad 6g
- Tangy Buffalo Best Chicken Wings 7g
- House Salad 9g
- Mediterranean Salad 9g
- Chicken Rustica 10g
- Side Caesar Salad 12g
- Tomato Basil Bliss Soup 16g
- Old Chicago Chopped Salad 23g
- Grilled Chicken Wrap With Lite Ranch 24g

Olive Garden

- Add Grilled Shrimp 0g
- Add Grilled Chicken 0g
- Italian Sausage 1g
- Parmesan Roasted Asparagus 3g
- Herb-Grilled Salmon (Dinner) 4g
- Low Fat Parmesan Peppercorn Dressing 5g
- Alfredo Dipping Sauce 5g
- Center Cut Filet Mignon 7g
- Sausage Pomodoro 8g
- Baked Tilapia With Shrimp 8g
- Chicken Meatballs 10g
- Garden-fresh Salad With Dressing 10g
- Grilled Chicken Caesar 10g
- Stuffed Mushrooms 12g
- Minestrone Soup 13g
- Mussels Di Napoli 13g
- Grilled Chicken Spiedini (Lunch) 19g
- All Chicken Mixed Grill (Gluten Free) 20g

On the Border Mexican Grill

- Savoy Pulled Pork (Carnitas) 0g
- House Salad No Dressing (Kid Side) 1g
- Pico de Gallo (Side) 1g
- Grilled Steak Mesquite 1g
- Mixed Cheese (Side) 1g
- Grilled Chicken 2g
- Hot Salsa 2g
- Chile Con Queso Without Chips (Cup) 7g
- Beef Crispy Taco 15g

Outback Steakhouse

- Joey Sirloin 0g
- Outback Center-Cut Sirloin (6 oz) 0g
- Ribeye (10 oz) 0g
- Sirloin 0g
- Joey Grilled Chicken On The Barbie 0g
- New York Strip (14 oz) 0g
- Victoria's Filet (7 oz) 0g
- Bushman Shrooms 0g
- Victoria's Filet (9 oz) 0g
- Prime Minister's Prime Rib 1g
- Kookaburra Wings - Hot 5g
- Crab Stuffed Shrimp (Aussie-tizer) 8g

P.F. Chang's China Bistro

- Gluten Free Spinach Stir-Fried with Garlic (Small) 1g
- Baby Steamed Buddha's Feast 3g
- Gluten Free Shanghai Cucumbers (Small) 4g
- Spinach Stir-Fried with Garlic (Small) 4g
- Teriyaki Sauce 5g
- Flaming Red Wontons 5g

- Wok-Seared Lamb 6g
- Northern Style Spare Ribs 6g
- Egg Drop Soup (cup) 6g
- Changs Vegetarian Lettuce Wraps 9g
- Hot and Sour soup (cup) 9g
- Chinese Chicken Lettuce Wraps 9g
- Gluten Free Chicken Lettuce Wraps 13g
- Wonton Soup (cup) 13g
- Edamame 13g

Panda Express

- Hot Mustard Sauce 0g
- Chili Sauce 2g
- Potsticker Sauce 3g
- Super Greens 5g
- Mixed Vegetables (Entree) 5g
- Kung Pao Sauce 6g
- Chinese Spare Ribs 6g
- Steamed Ginger Fish 8g
- Kung Pao Shrimp 10
- Five Flavor Shrimp (Small) 13g
- Wok Fired Shrimp 18g
- Wok-Seared Steak & Shrimp 20g

Panera Bread

- Greek Salad (Half) 4g
- Power Mediterranean Chicken Salad 7g
- Chopped Chicken Cobb Salad 8g
- Grilled Chicken Caesar Salad (Half) 9g
- Asian Sesame Chicken Salad (Half) 11g
- Mediterranean Salmon Salad (Half) 12g
- Fuji Apple Chicken Salad (Half) 14g

Papa John's Pizza

- Special Garlic Dipping Sauce 0g
- Unsauced Roasted Wings 0g
- Crushed Red Pepper 1g
- Ranch Dipping Sauce 1g
- Blue Cheese Dipping Sauce 1g
- 8 Wings With No Sauce 4g
- Chicken Strips 10g

Papa Murphy's Take 'N' Bake

- Low Calorie Italian Salad Dressing 1g
- Marinara Sauce (Cup) 2g
- Caesar Salad 2g
- Buttermilk Ranch Salad Dressing 2g
- Chicken Caesar Salad 2g
- Club Salad 3g
- Chicken Bacon Artichoke Crustless 3g
- Italian Salad 4g
- Garden Salad 5g
- Gourmet Supreme DeLITE Thin Crust Pizza (Large) 13g
- Mediterranean Salad 14g
- Chicken Caesar Salad 17g

Peet's Coffee and Tea

- Toasted Almonds 1g
- Egg & Cheddar Breakfast Sandwich (No Bun) 4g
- Maple Chicken Sausage (No Bun) 4g
- Bacon, Spinach & Swiss Quiche 10g
- Market Box 11g
- Wild Blueberries 13g
- Chocolate Toffee Almonds 21g

Pei Wei Asian Kitchen

- Vietnamese Black Pepper Slaw 6g

- Spring Roll 1g
- Cauliflower Rice (Small) 1g
- Crab Wontons 12g
- Thai Dynamite Shrimp 18g
- Mongolian Shrimp 18g
- Ginger Broccoli with Shrimp 16g
- Thai Coconut Curry Beef 18
- Mandarin Kung Pao Shrimp 21g
- Spicy Korean Shrimp 21g
- Thai Coconut Curry Chicken 21g
- Sesame Shrimp 25g

Perkins Restaurant & Bakery

- Monterey Jack Cheese 0g
- Fresh Broccoli 0g
- Fresh Mushrooms 0g
- Shredded Monterey Jack and Swiss Cheddar Cheese 0g
- Fresh Asparagus 0g
- Fresh Spinach 0g
- Applewood Smoked Bacon (1 Slice) 0g
- Patties Sausage (2) 1g
- Grilled Pork Chops 2g
- Chicken & Spinach Salad 6g
- Deli Ham & Cheese Omelette 8g
- Chef's Salad 13g
- Glazed Baby Carrots 13g

Peter Piper Pizza

- Chef Salad 12g
- Italian Chef Salad 12g
- Mandarin Cranberry Salad (Small) 21g
- Original Crust Pepperoni Pizza 1 Slice (Large) 34g
- Chicago Classic Pizza (Large) 1 Slice 36g

Pizza Hut

- Baked Mild/Hot Wings 1g
- Wing Dipping Sauce - Ranch 2g
- Bone Out Wings - All American Wings 10g
- Grilled Chicken Salad 14g
- Medium Meat Lover's Thin'N Crispy Pizza (1 Slice) 22g

Pizza Ranch

- Chicken Leg 2g
- Broasted Chicken Wing 2g
- Broasted Chicken Breast 4g
- Broasted Chicken Thigh 4g
- Potato Wedges 13g
- Pepperoni Pizza 20g
- Bronco Pizza 23g
- Cheese Pizza 24g

Pollo Tropical

- Boneless Chicken Breasts (6 oz) 0g
- Grilled Tropical Wings 0g
- 1/4 Chicken Dark Meat 0g
- Boneless Chicken Breast (4 oz) 0g
- Curry Mustard Sauce 0g
- 1/4 Chicken White Meat 0g
- 1/2 Chicken 0g
- 1/4 Rack Ribs 1g

Popeyes Louisiana Kitchen

- Mild Chicken Leg (Skinless & Breading Removed) 0g
- Mild Chicken Thigh (Skinless & Breading Removed) 0g
- Mild Chicken Breast (Skinless & Breading Removed) 0g
- Spicy Chicken Wing (Skinless & Breading Removed) 0g
- Spicy Chicken Leg (Skinless & Breading Removed) 0g
- Spicy Chicken Breast (Skinless & Breading Removed) 0g
- Tartar Sauce 1g
- Blackened Ranch Sauce 2g
- Blackened Tenders 2g
- Chicken Etouffee (Side) 4g
- Green Beans 5g
- Mild Chicken Thigh 6g
- Spicy Chicken Wing 7g
- Mild Chicken Breast 8g
- Nuggets (6 Piece) 13g

Portillo's

- Bacon Burger (No Bun) 4g
- Chopped Salad (No Pasta) 6g
- Italian Beef (No Bread) 6g
- House Dressing 6g
- Chicago Combo Bowl 6g
- Chicken Pecan Salad 8g
- Classic Beef Bowl 9g
- Cup of Cheese Sauce 10g
- Garden Salad (No Dressing) 10g
- Grilled Chicken Sandwich 1g

Potbelly Sandwich Shop

- Pickle 1g
- Hot Peppers 2g
- Buttermilk Ranch Dressing 4g
- Hummus 6g

- Bacon, Egg & Cheddar Square (No Bread) 6g
- Farmhouse Salad 7g
- Wreck Salad 8g
- Roasted Garlic Vinaigrette 10g
- Spicy Black Bean & Roasted Tomato Soup 1g
- Garden Vegetable Soup (Cup) 12g
- The Powerhouse 12g

Pret A Manger

- Egg & Spinach Pot 1g
- Chicken, Smoked Bacon & Avocado Salad 2g
- Balsamic Vinaigrette 2g
- Tahini Yogurt Dressing 2g
- Coconut Greens Dressing 2g
- Simple Tuna Salad 2g
- Lemon Shallot Dressing 2g
- Chicken & Edamame Protein Pot 3g
- Low Fat Yogurt, Blueberry & Granola PretPot 8g
- The Royal Chef Salad 8g
- Wild Salmon Salad 10g
- Italian Meat Soup 18g

Qdoba Mexican Eats

- Bacon 0g
- Mexican Caesar Dressing 1g
- Grilled Chicken 1g
- Three Cheese Queso 2g
- Pico de Gallo 2g
- Cilantro Lime Dressing 2g
- Chicken 2g
- Smoked Brisket 3g
- Grill Steak 3g
- Mexican Cauliflower Mash 6g

- Grill Naked Chicken Taco Salad 7g
- Pulled Pork 10g
- Naked Chicken Taco Salad (No Dressing) 13g
- Cauli-Mash Low-Carb Chicken Bowl 22g

Raising Cane's Chicken Fingers

- Naked Bird 0g
- Chicken Fingers 5g
- Cane's Sauce 6g
- Coleslaw 10g
- Chicken Tenders 18g

Rally's Hamburgers

- Bacon Cheddar Burger (No Bun, No Ketchup) 2g
- All American Cheeseburger (No Bun, No Ketchup) 2g
- Cheese Double Cheese (No Bun) 2g
- Chili Dog (No Bun, No Chili) 2g
- Spicy Chicken Sandwich (No Bun) 8g
- Crispy Fish Sandwich (No Bun) 20g

Red Lobster

- Crab Crackin' Monday (1 Pound) 0g
- Chilled Jumbo Shrimp Cocktail 0g
- Petite Shrimp Salad Topping 0g
- Red Snapper 0g
- Unsweetened Iced Tea or Hot Tea 0g
- Center - Cut NY Strip Steak 0g
- Snow Crab Legs (1 Pound) 0g
- Wood-Grilled Or Broiled Tilapia (Half Portion) 8g

Red Robin Gourmet Burgers

- Burger Patty 0g
- Beef Patty 0g

- Bleu Cheese Dressing 0g
- Chick On A Stick 0g
- Turkey Burger Patty 1g
- Iced Tea 1g
- Ranch Dressing 1g
- Lettuce Wrapped Protein Burger 6g

Romano's Macaroni Grill

- Romano's Macaroni Grill Center-Cut Filet: 14g
- Romano's Macaroni Grill Chicken Caesar Salad: 15g
- Romano's Macaroni Grill Chicken Under A Brick: 18g
- Romano's Macaroni Grill Grilled Asparagus (Side): 2g
- Romano's Macaroni Grill Grilled Chicken & Broccoli: 15g
- Romano's Macaroni Grill Handmade Meatballs: 13g
- Romano's Macaroni Grill King Salmon Spiedini: 22g
- Romano's Macaroni Grill Mediterranean Olives: 2g
- Romano's Macaroni Grill Sauteed Shrimp: 0g
- Romano's Macaroni Grill Scallops & Spinach Salad (Zuppa Della Casa & Insalata): 12g

Round Table Pizza

- Honey BBQ Wings 2g
- Pepperoni Original Pizza (Personal) 15g
- Cheese Pizza (Personal) 15g
- Guinevere's Garden Delight (Personal) 16g
- Maui Zaui Skinny Crust Pizza (Large) 19g
- Montague's All Meat Marvel 22g
- Pepperoni Original Pizza (Large) 23g
- Wombo Combo Original Pizza (Large) 24g

Rubio's Coastal Grill

- Pan Seared Shrimp 0g
- Carnitas Street Taco 6g
- Chicken Street Taco 6g

- Chicken Fiesta Salad (No Dressing) 7g
- Steak Street Taco 9g
- Chopped Salad 14g
- Steak Taco 19g
- Grill Carnitas Taco 20g
- Balsamic & Roasted Veggie Salad 20g
- Grill Salsa Verde Shrimp Taco 21g
- Grill Fish Taco 23g

Ruby Tuesday

- Lobster Entree 0g
- Lobster Tail Add-On 0g
- Fire Wings 0g
- Skinny Lavender Lemon Drop 0g
- Blackened Tilapia 0g
- Grilled Salmon 0g
- Creole Catch 0g
- Plain Grilled Top Sirloin 0g
- Lobster Entree 0g
- Fresh Steamed Broccoli 3g
- Side Of Premium Baby Green Beans 5g
- New Orleans Seafood 6g
- Memphis Dry Rub Half-Rack Ribs 6g
- Top Sirloin 9g
- Buffalo Shrimp 11g
- Chicken Strips - Thai Phoon 12g
- Memphis Dry Rub Full-Rack Ribs 12g
- Grilled Chicken Salad 15g
- Jumbo Lump Crab Cake 16g

Ruth's Chris Steak House

- T-Bone 0g
- Petite Filet Shrimp 0g
- Porterhouse 0g

- New York Steak 0g
- Cowboy Ribeye 0g
- Petite Filet Mignon 0g
- Cream Cheese Stuffed Chicken Breast 6g
- Steak House Salad 6g
- Creamed Spinach 14g

Saltgrass Steak House

- Any Solo Steak Option 1g
- Hickory Chicken Breast 4g
- Caesar Side Salad 4g
- Steak Salad 10g

Sarku Japan

- Miso Soup 6g
- Chicken Teriyaki (No Rice, No Sauce) 6g
- Seaweed Salad 13g

Sbarro

- Vodka Sauce 4g
- Marinara Sauce 4g
- Mixed Garden Salad 4g
- Caesar Dressing 5g
- Caesar Salad 5g
- Chicken Portofino 6g
- Chicken Francese 6g
- Chicken Vesuvio 7g
- Cucumber & Tomato Salad 7g
- Meatballs 9g
- Chicken Parmesan 14g
- Low Carb Cheese Pizza 14g
- Low Carb Sausage & Pepperoni Pizza 14g
- Sausage & Peppers 15g

Schlotzsky's

- Baby Spinach & Feta Salad 3g
- Hearty Vegetable Beef Soup (Bowl) 8g
- Garden Salad 8g
- Broccoli Cheese Soup (Cup) 12g
- Chicken Tortilla Soup (Cup) 12g
- Turkey Chef Salad 13g

Seasons 52

- Organic Mixed Greens (with Sunflower Seeds) 4g
- Organic Portobello Salad 7g
- Tandoori Chicken Skewers 8g
- Blackened Fish Tacos 1g
- Kalymnos Greek Salad 1g
- Crab & Shrimp Stuffed Mushrooms 12g
- Shrimp & Chicken Gumbo (8 oz) 13g
- Flat Iron Steak Salad 17g
- Grilled Rack Of New Zealand Lamb 17g
- Wood-Roasted Pork Tenderloin 25g

Shake Shack

- Shack Sauce 0g
- Lettuce Wrap 0g
- Bacon (2 Slices) 0g
- American Cheese 1g
- Shack Burger (No Bun) 2g
- Seasonal Fresh Fruit Topping 3g
- Double Cheeseburger (No Bun) 5g

- Chick'n Shack (No Bun) 5g
- Peanut Butter Topping 8g
- Chocolate Truffle Cookie Dough Topping 10g
- Chick'N Bites 18g

Sharis

- Shari's Spring Spinach Omelet 8 Carbs
- Shari's BMP Omelet 8 Carbs
- Shari's Chicken Fajita Omelet 9 Carbs
- Shari's Denver Omelet 10 Carbs

Sheetz

- MTO Burger (No Bun) 0g
- Fried Egg Patty 1g
- Mild Pepper Rings 1g
- Scrambled Egg Patty 1g
- Pepper Jack Cheese 2g
- Mild Cheddar Cheese 2g
- Italian Meat Combo 2g
- Grilled Chicken Caesar Salad 4g
- Natural Pistachios 4g
- Italian Salad 4g
- Wisconsin Cheese Bites (Regular) 8g
- Veggie Snack 8g
- Beef & Cheddar Snack Tray 12g
- Grilled Chicken Wrap 14g
- Chef Salad 15g
- Omelet Wrap 15g

Shoney's

- Smoked Sausage Sliced 3g
- Scrambled Eggs 3g
- Stewed Tomatoes No Salt Added 5g

- Creamy Peanut Butter 2 tbsp
- Fried Chicken Leg 6g
- Green Beans 7g
- Cheese (Salad Bar) 8g
- All American Burger (No Bun) 10g
- Thin Crust Firehouse Pizza (Large) 18g

Sizzler

- Grilled Salmon 0g
- Ranch Dressing 1g
- Greek Salad 1g
- Taco Meat 1g
- Tuna Pasta Salad 1g
- Steak (6 oz) 2g
- Italian Dressing 2g
- Chicken Wings 2g
- Italian Herb Chicken 3g
- Double Hibachi Chicken 9g
- Broccoli Cheese Soup 10g
- Seafood Salad 1g
- Malibu Chicken (Single) 1g

Smashburger

- Bacon 0g
- Big Smash Patty 1g
- Grilled Onions 1g
- Smash Sauce 1g
- Regular Beef Patty 1g
- Ranch Dressing 1g
- Grilled Chicken Breast 1g
- Side Salad (No Dressing) 2g
- Baja Cobb Salad (Regular) 6g
- Crispy Brussel Sprouts 9g
- Chicken Strips With Ranch 13g

- Avocado Club Smashchicken 25g

Smokey Bones Bar & Fire Grill

- 7 oz Top Sirloin Blue Cheese with 0g
- Grouper Grilled Entree with 1g
- Fresh Steamed Broccoli with 2g
- 7 oz Top Sirloin with Mushroom Sauce with 3g
- Flame Seared Salmon with 4g
- Caesar Side Salad with 6g
- Chicken Caesar Salad with 6g
- Grouper Blackened Entree with 6g
- Garden Green Side Salad with 7g
- Smokey Bones Teriyaki Salmon 9g
- Smokey Bones Smoked St. Louis Ribs (1/3 Rack) 17g
- Smokey Bones Hand Pulled Pork 17g

Smoothie King

- Gladiator Smoothie (32 oz) 1g
- Gladiator Smoothie (40 oz) 1g
- Gladiator Protein 1g
- Vegetable Mix 1g
- Gladiator Chocolate 4g
- Low Carb Chocolate Smoothie (20 oz) 6g
- Keto Champ Coffee (20 oz) 7g
- Low Carb Chocolate Smoothie (32 Oz) 9g
- Skinny High Protein Smoothie - Chocolate (20 Oz) 17g

Sonic Drive-in

- Bacon 0g
- Cheeseburger (No Bun) 0g
- String Cheese 0g
- Mozzarella Sticks (1 Oz) 4g
- Chili Cheese Coney (No Bun) 4g

- Grilled Chicken Salad 9g
- Chicken Strips (Kids Meal) 9g
- Chicken Strips (3) 14g

Sonny's BBQ

- 1/4 Bar-B-Q Chicken 0g
- 1/2 Bar-B-Q Chicken 0g
- Whole Bar-B-Q Chicken 0g
- Sliced Pork (Lunch) 1g
- Sliced Pork (Dinner) 1g
- Charbroiled Chicken (Lunch) 1g
- Pulled Chicken (Lunch) 1g
- Bar-B-Q Chicken & Sliced Pork 1g
- Broccoli 3g
- Smoked Turkey (Lunch) 4g
- Southern Green Beans 7g
- Big Salad With Sliced Beef 27g

Starbucks Coffee

- Protein & Fiber Powder 0g
- Caffe Americano (Short) 1g
- Mixed Nuts 2g
- Whipped Cream Topping 2g
- Turkey & Swiss Sandwich (No Bun) 4g
- Ham, Egg Frittata, Cheddar Cheese (No Roll) 4g
- Skinny Vanilla Latte (Short) 9g
- Farmer's Market Salad 19g

Steak 'n Shake

- Sausage Patty 0g
- Iced Tea (Unsweetened) 0g

- Breakfast Bowl Without Hash Browns 4g
- Double Steakburger (No Bun) 4g
- Small Garden Salad 7g
- Cottage Cheese With Pineapple Ring 10g
- Cheddar Scrambler 10g
- Vegetable Soup (Cup) 10g
- Frisco Steakburger 14g
- BBQ Steakburger 16g
- Chicken Gumbo Soup (Bowl) 19g

Subway

- Pepper Jack Cheese 0g
- Chicken Strips 0g
- Vinegar 0g
- Mozzarella Cheese Shredded 0g
- Jalapeno Peppers 0g
- Banana Peppers 0g
- Cheddar Cheese 0g
- Black Olives 0g
- Swiss Cheese 0g
- Roasted Chicken Patty 4g
- Oven Roasted Chicken Breast Salad 6g
- Turkey Breast Salad 8g
- Cold Cut Combo Protein Bowl 8g
- Chicken & Bacon Ranch Protein Bowl 11g
- Turkey 'Cali Fresh' Protein Bowl 12g

Taco Bell

- Mini Skillet Bowl (No Potato/Add Meat) 5g
- Beefy 5-Layer Burrito Bowl (No Tortilla/No Beans) 6g
- Power Menu Bowl (No Rice/Beans) 6g
- Grande Scrambler Burrito Bowl (No Potatoes) 7g
- Fiesta Taco Salad with Chicken 10g

Taco Cabana

- Bacon 0g
- Scrambled Egg 0g
- Salsa Roja (1 oz) 1g
- Salsa Verde (1 oz) 1g
- Salsa Fuego (1 oz) 1g
- Salsa Ranch (1 oz) 1g
- Pico De Gallo 1g
- Southwest Ranch Dressing (1 oz) 2g
- Crispy Chicken Taco 1g
- Chicken Taco Stewed Chicken 1g
- Shrimp Enchilada 16g
- Steak & Egg Taco 20g

Taco John's

- Side Salad 2g
- House Dressing 2g
- Nacho Cheese 5g
- Crispy Taco 9g
- Shredded Beef Street Taco 15g
- Chicken Bacon Guac Street Taco 16g
- Chicken Street Taco 16g
- Chicken Snack Quesadilla 17g

Texas Roadhouse

- Oven Roasted Chicken Quarter 0g
- Sirloin Kabob 0g
- Dallas Fillet (6 oz) 0g
- Ribeye (6 oz) 0g
- New York Strip Steak (12 oz) 0g
- Ribeye (10 oz) 0g
- Grilled Pork Chop 0g

- Road Kill 4g
- Cinnamon Butter 5g
- Grilled Chicken Salad 10g
- Portobello Mushroom Chicken 1g
- Grilled Salmon 17g

TGI Fridays

- Sizzling Sirloin & Spinach 0g
- Bacon Cheddar Beef Patties 2g
- Flat Iron Steak 2g
- Spinach, Cheese & Artichoke Dip 2g
- Buffalo Wing Sauce 2g
- Petite Sirloin 2g
- Queso Dip 2g
- Original Flavor Steak Strips 3g
- Fresh Vegetable Medley 4g
- Sizzling Chicken & Spinach 5g
- Grilled Chicken Cobb Salad 10g
- Mozzarella Sticks 10g
- Boneless Buffalo Chicken Bites 15g
- Sizzling Chicken & Broccoli 15g
- TGI Boneless Chicken Bites Honey BBQ Style Sauce 16g

The Capital Grilleburger

- Bone-In Dry Aged Strip 14 oz 0g
- Filet Mignon 8 oz 2g
- Boneless Ribeye 14 oz 4g
- Wedge Salad With Blue Cheese & Bacon 8g
- Lobster Bisque - Cup 10g
- New England Clam Chowder - Cup 13g

The Cheesecake Factory

- Tropical Iced Tea 4g

- Crab Cakes with 6g of net carbs
- 6 Carb Original Cheesecake 6g
- Ahi Tartare 8g
- Skinnylicious Mexican Chicken Lettuce Wrap Tacos 9g
- Tortilla Soup 9g
- Steak Diane Without Mashed Potatoes 10g
- Skinnylicious Asian Chicken Lettuce Wraps 1g
- Tuscan Chicken 14

The Habit Burger Grill

- Seasoned Beef Patty 0g
- Bacon with 0g of net carbs
- Blue Cheese Dressing 1g
- Chunky Avocado 1g
- American Cheese 1g
- Bacon (2 strips): 0g
- Seasoned, Grilled Beef Patty: 0g
- Seasoned, Grilled Chicken Breast 2g
- Ranch Dressing 2g
- Seasoned, Grilled Chicken Breast 2g
- House Dressing 3g
- Grilled Chicken Salad 5g
- Seasoned, Grilled Tenderloin Steak 6g
- Side Salad (No Dressing) 7g
- Seasoned, Chargrilled Ahi Tuna 7g
- Santa Barbara Cobb Salad 8g

The Melting Pot

- Breast of Chicken - Mojo 0g
- Land & Sea, Coq au Vin 2g
- Vegetable Cup for Cheese Fondue 3g
- California Salad 3g
- Spinach Mushroom Salad 4g
- Cheddar Cheese Fondue 7g

- Fiesta Cheese Fondue 8g
- Traditional Swiss Cheese Fondue 9g
- Cut Apples for Cheese Fondue 15g

Tim Hortons

- Herb & Garlic Cream Cheese 2g
- Plain Cream Cheese 2g
- Light Plain Cream Cheese 2g
- Garden Vegetable Cream Cheese 3g
- Bacon & Cheese Omelette Bites 3g
- Spinach & Egg White Omelette Bites 3g
- Old Fashioned Plain Cake Timbits 5g
- Old Fashioned Plain Timbit 7g
- Egg & Cheese Wrap 15g
- Sausage Breakfast Wrap 16g
- Chicken Ranch Wrap 20g

Tropical Smoothie Cafe

- Whey Protein 2g
- Whey Protein Supplement 2g
- Pea Protein 4g
- Beach Club Salad 7g
- Chicken Caesar Salad 7g
- Kale & Apple Slaw 9g
- Buffalo Chicken Bowl 12g
- Smoked Jalapeño Chicken Taco 16g
- Cranberry Walnut Chicken Salad 17g
- Thai Chili Steak Taco 22g

True Food Kitchen

- Organic Tuscan Kale Salad 8g
- Roasted Brussel Sprouts 13g
- Sweet Potato Hash 15g

- Cauliflower Polenta Bowl 21g
- Butternut Squash Soup 21g
- Lasagna Bolognese 26g
- Edamame Dumplings 29g

Twin Peaks

- Protein Puffs Jalapeño Cheddar 2g
- Protein Puffs 2g
- Protein Puffs Nacho Cheese 2g
- House Salad 9g
- Crispy Buffalo Chicken Salad 35g

Uno Chicago Grillpizzeria Uno

- Kid's Grilled Chicken 0g
- 8 oz Top Sirloin 0g
- Steak on A Stick 0g
- 10 oz Top Sirloin 0g
- The Chop House Classic 0g
- 6 oz Top Sirloin 0g
- 7 oz Filet Mignon 0g
- Grilled Shrimp And Sirloin 1g
- Chicken Gorgonzola 1g
- Grill Grilled Rosemary Chicken 1g
- Three Way Buffalo Wings 3g
- Steamed Seasonal Vegetables 6g
- Gorgonzola Walnut Side Salad 8g
- House Side Salad 8g
- French Onion Soup 12g
- Shrimp And Crab Fondue 13g

Village Inn

- Sausage Patty 0g
- Sausage Links 0g
- 2 Bacon Strips 0g
- Sausage Links 0g
- 2 Egg Cheese Omelet 1g
- 2 Eggs, Any Style Except Poached 1g
- Ranch Dressing 2g
- 2 Egg White Omelet with Part-Skim Mozzarella 2g
- Lemon Artichoke Chicken (No Side) 5g
- Side Garden Salad (No Dressing) 5g
- Tomato Basil Soup 5g
- Fruit Cup 6g
- Chicken Noodle Soup 10g
- Avocado Swiss Chicken 11g
- Cobb Salad 12g

Waffle House

- Sausage Patties (2) 0g
- Sirloin Steak 0g
- Bacon 0g
- Grilled Plain Chicken Breast 0g
- Pork Chop 0g
- Bacon (3) 0g
- Country Ham 0g
- Cheese & Eggs 1g
- Sautéed Onions 2g
- Cheesesteak Omelet 5g
- Fiesta Omelet 7g
- Ham & Cheese Omelet 10g

Wawa

- Egg 1g
- Diet Green Tea (Bottle) with 1g of net carbs
- Diet Iced Tea Lemon with 1g of net carbs

- Diet Lemonade Tea with 2g of net carbs
- Premium Oven Roasted Turkey with 2g
- Exp Roasted Chicken Salad 6g
- Scrambled Egg Bowl 9g
- Scrambled Egg Bowl With Turkey Sausage 10g
- Caribbean Style Chicken Salad 17g

Wendy's

- 1/4 Lb Hamburger Patty 0g
- Grilled Chicken Fillet 1g
- Cheesy Cheddarburger (No Bun) 1g
- Double Stack (No Bun) 2g
- Caesar Side Salad (No Croutons) 3g
- Ultimate Chicken Grill (No Bun) 6g
- Chicken BLT Salad (No Dressing & Croutons) 8g
- Chicken BLT Salad (No Dressing) 16g

Wetzel's

- Cheese Dog (No Bun) 1g

Whataburger

- Double Meat Whataburger (No Bun) 3g
- Mushroom Swiss Burger (No Bun)
- Monterey Melt (No Bun) 5g
- Garden Salad With Grilled Chicken 6g
- Chicken Strip (1 Piece) 10g
- Grilled Chicken Salad 12g

Which Wich Superior Sandwiches

- Chicken 0g
- Pepper Jack Cheese 0g
- Pork Tenderloin 0g

- Provolone Cheese 0g
- Blue Cheese 0g
- Chicken Pesto 0g
- Corned Beef 0g
- American Cheese 0g
- French Dip Meat 1g
- Egg 2g
- Sausage & Egg 2g
- Bac-Hammon 2g
- Crab Salad 15g

White Castle

- Sausage 0g
- Strip Of Bacon 0g
- Egg 1g
- Double White Castle (No Bun) 1g
- Hamburger & Egg Sandwich (No Bun) 1g
- Chicken Rings (3) 8g
- Clam Strips (Regular) 5g
- Chicken Rings (6) 12g
- Savory Grilled Chicken Slider 12g
- Bacon Jalapeno Cheeseburger 14g

Wienerschnitzel

- Side Salad 1g
- Italian Dressing 1g
- Ranch Dressing 2g
- Sandwich with Egg, Bacon & Cheese (No Bun) 2g
- Chili Cheeseburger (No Bun) 7g
- Corn Dog 14g
- Jalapeno Poppers (3 Pack) 19g
- Mini Corn Dogs (6-Pack) 21g

Wingstop

- Cajun Wings with 0g
- Boneless Wings with 0g
- Regular Mild Wings 0g
- Lemon Pepper Wings 0g
- Original Hot Wings 0g
- Plain Jumbo Wings 0g
- Louisiana Rub Wings 0g
- Garlic Parmesan Wings 0g
- Ranch Dip 2g
- Blue Cheese 3g
- Veggie Sticks 7g

Yard House

- Ranch Dressing 1g
- Grilled Chicken Caesar Salad 4g
- Caesar Salad 5g
- Ahi Caesar Salad 5g
- Black Truffle Cheeseburger (No Bun) 7g
- Edamame (Half) 8g
- Roasted Turkey Cobb Salad 9g
- Seared Ahi Sashimi 12g
- French Onion Soup (Cup) 14g

Zaxby's

- Grilled Chicken Breast 0g
- Unsweetened Tea (22 oz) 0g
- Buffalo Wings 0g
- Unsweetened Tea (12 oz) 0g
- Unsweetened Tea (32 oz) 0g
- Traditional Wings (5) 0g
- Blackened Blue Zalad (No Bread) 9g
- Buffalo Chicken Fingerz (10)
- Chicken Fingerz (5) 12g

Zoes Kitchen

- Chicken Salad (Side) 1g
- Salmon Kabob 2g
- Shrimp Kabob 3g
- Chicken Kabob 4g
- Marinated Slaw 4g
- Grilled Chicken 5g
- Mediterranean Lamb Kafta 6g
- Protein Power Plate 1g
- Grilled Chicken Salad 16g

Printed in Great Britain
by Amazon